Joint Commission
RESOURCES

PROTECTING THOSE WHO SERVE:

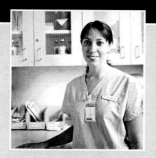 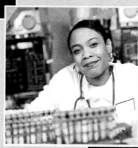 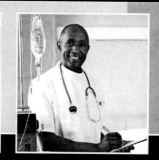

Health Care Worker Safety

Improving Health Care Quality and Safety

Joint Commission Resources Mission

The mission of Joint Commission Resources is to continuously improve the safety and quality of care in the United States and in the international community through the provision of education and consultation services and international accreditation.

Joint Commission Resources educational programs and publications support, but are separate from, the accreditation activities of the Joint Commission. Attendees at Joint Commission Resources educational programs and purchasers of Joint Commission Resources publications receive no special consideration or treatment in, or confidential information about, the accreditation process.

The inclusion of an organization name, product, or service in a Joint Commission publication should not be construed as an endorsement of such organization, product, or service, nor is failure to include an organization name, product, or service to be construed as disapproval.

This publication is designed to provide accurate and authoritative information regarding the subject matter covered. Every attempt has been made to ensure accuracy at the time of publication; however, please note that laws, regulations, and standards are subject to change. Please also note that some of the examples in this publication are specific to the laws and regulations of the locality of the facility. The information and examples in this publication are provided with the understanding that the publisher is not engaged in providing medical, legal, or other professional advice. If any such assistance is desired, the services of a competent professional person should be sought.

© 2005 by the Joint Commission on Accreditation of Healthcare Organizations

Joint Commission Resources, Inc. (JCR), a not-for-profit affiliate of the Joint Commission on Accreditation of Healthcare Organizations (Joint Commission), has been designated by the Joint Commission to publish publications and multimedia products. JCR reproduces and distributes these materials under license from the Joint Commission.

All rights reserved. No part of this publication may be reproduced in any form or by any means without written permission from the publisher.

Printed in the U.S.A. 5 4 3 2 1

ISBN: 0-86688-920-5

LCCN: 2005923340

For more information about Joint Commission Resources, please visit http://www.jcrinc.com.

Senior Editor:
Kristine M. Miller, M.F.A.

Project Manager:
Christine Wyllie

Manager, Publications:
Diane Bell

Production Manager:
Johanna Harris

Associate Director:
Cecily Pew

Executive Director:
Catherine Chopp Hinckley, Ph.D.

Vice President, Publications:
George J. Farina

Joint Commission Reviewers:
George Mills, F.A.S.H.E, C.H.F.M., C.E.M., *Associate Director, Standards Interpretation Group*;
Dave Kitchin, FACHE, FHFI, CHE, *JCR consultant*

OSHA Reviewers:
Don Wright, M.D., M.P.H., *Director, Office of Occupational Medicine*;
Patricia A. Bray, M.D., M.P.H., *Medical Officer*;
Kay A. Dellinger, M.D., M.P.H, *Medical Officer*;
Atkinson W. (Jack) Longmire, M.D., *Medical Officer*;
John D. Piacentino, M.D., M.P.H., *Medical Officer*;
Angela C. Presson, M.D., M.P.H., *Medical Officer*

Requests for permission to make copies of any part of this work should be mailed to:

Permissions Editor
Department of Publications
Joint Commission Resources
One Renaissance Boulevard
Oakbrook Terrace, Illinois 60181
permissions@jcrinc.com

TABLE OF CONTENTS

Introduction
The Joint Commission and OSHA:
An Educational Partnership 2
Joint Commission Standards
and Employee Safety..........................2
Survey/Inspection Activity 2
Content of the Book...........................2
Important Distinctions 3
Frequently Used Terms 3

CHAPTER ONE:
OSHA Programs and Joint Commission Standards
Safety and Health Programs 7
Using a Matrix to Identify Areas
for Improvement 12
Applying Results Across the System ..13
Using Education to Ensure Safety 14
Commitment to Culture of Safety 14
Voluntary Protection Programs 16
Working Toward the Goal 16
Building on Success 17
Achieving the Goal 18
Hazard Communication (HAZCOM) ..18
OSHA Recordkeeping and 300 Log ..21
Conclusion 22

CHAPTER TWO:
Facility-Related Risks
Confined Space 25
Fire Safety 26
Control of Hazardous Energy and
Electrical Safety 28
Ventilation 30
Why Address Mold? 38
Creating the Program 38
Program Content 38
Implementing the Program 39
Asbestos...40
Hearing Conservation.......................42
Machine Guarding 44
Conclusion 47

CHAPTER THREE:
Human Factor-Related Risks
Violence Prevention in the Workplace ..49
Ergonomics 60
Investing in Infrastructure 65
Adapting to the Acute Care Environment..65
Winning over the Hospital Nurse 68
High-end Technology, Quick ROI 68
Emergency Action Planning.............68
Personal Protective Equipment 71
Respiratory Protection 79
Conclusion 84

CHAPTER FOUR:
Clinically Related Risks
Bloodborne Pathogens 87
Tuberculosis......................................93
Legionella 97
Ethylene Oxide, Formaldehyde,
and Glutaraldehyde 103
Hazardous Drugs, Reproductive Hazards,
and Anesthetic Gas..........................107
Conclusion 112

CHAPTER FIVE:
Performance Measurement and Worker Safety
Performance Monitoring in
the Environment of Care 116
The Joint Commission and
Performance Improvement.............119
Putting It All Together 119

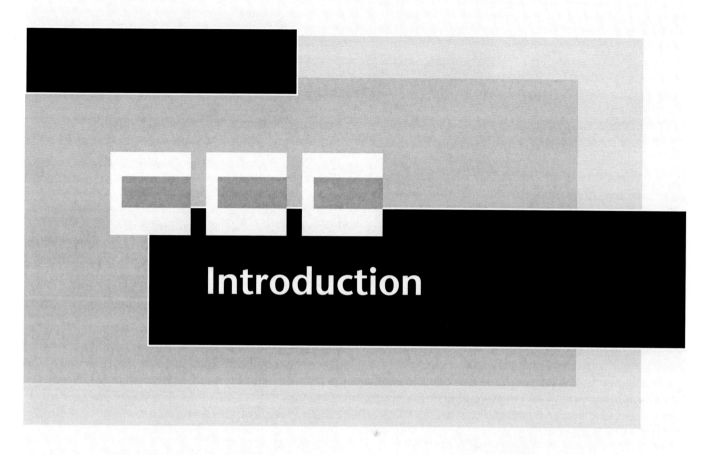

Introduction

HEALTH CARE WORKERS may be health care's single most important asset. Without the health care worker, patient care cannot occur. Yet according to Bureau of Labor Statistics, more than 500,000 heath care workers suffer work-related injuries annually, including back injuries, plus injuries associated with fire, hazardous chemicals, electrical issues, and other risks.[1] Last year alone an estimated 800,000 accidental needlesticks occurred in hospital settings, putting health care workers at risk for exposure to various bloodborne pathogens.

Who is responsible for overall safety in a health care organization? Is it the safety officer? administration? department directors and managers? the front line supervisors? The answer to all these questions is yes, and more. *Everyone* is responsible for safety. It is a responsibility throughout the organization.

While the safety officer (or a team of several individuals) typically serves as the manager of the overall safety process, he or she alone is not responsible for safety. Typically the safety officer is a resource person to whom others in the organization may direct questions about regulatory compliance, request approval of policies and procedures, and from whom they may seek guidance. He or she may coordinate the development, implementation, and monitoring of safety management activities.

The administration and leadership of an organization play a critical role in the safety of the organization's members. It is important for leadership to value, commit to, and support safe work practices in an organization for safety to permeate the culture. Organization leaders should set expectations that staff will always work safely and follow all the pertinent safety rules. Leadership must also "walk the talk." Staff members will not focus on safety if leadership does not.

Department directors, managers, and supervisors are responsible for the development of department-specific safety policies and organizationwide safety policies as well as the enforcement of these policies. They are the people who make the daily observations of staff member performance and provide ongoing coaching as well as annual performance assessments. These individuals are key to the effectiveness of the safety culture because they expect safety from their staff members as well as of themselves.

Staff are also responsible for safety, particularly in their daily workplace activities. While staff can take short cuts around the safety rules due to workload constraints, inattention, or simply because it's easier, health care workers must demand more from themselves and always do it the right way: the safe way.

THE JOINT COMMISSION AND OSHA: AN EDUCATIONAL PARTNERSHIP

The Occupational Safety and Health Administration (OSHA) is a government agency dedicated to ensuring the safety and health of America's workers by setting and enforcing standards; providing training, outreach, and education; establishing partnerships; and encouraging continual improvement in workplace safety and health. In 1996, the Joint Commission and OSHA, recognizing their complementary goals regarding safety, teamed up in an educational partnership. The goals of this partnership are to foster improvement in management of safety and health issues in health care organizations and minimize duplication in compliance activities between the two organizations.

The partnership between OSHA and the Joint Commission has been renewed several times over the years—most recently as of January 1, 2005. Throughout the years, the educational efforts of this partnership have focused on addressing and reducing the increasing number of health care worker illnesses and injuries. Educational efforts have specifically addressed the issue of biological and airborne hazards in health care as well as other safety concerns.

The Joint Commission's "Management of the Environment of Care" (EC) standards are very similar to OSHA's General Industry Standards.[2] For example, the seven Joint Commission EC management plans shown in Sidebar I-1 on this page are common to OSHA's Environment of Work concerns.[3]

The Joint Commission and OSHA share concerns about the strategies used to protect health care workers. Therefore, the organizations' standards and requirements both focus on ergonomics, bloodborne pathogen control, violence prevention, hazardous materials management, and life safety.[3] The overlap between the "environment of care" and the "environment of work" is shown in Figure I-1.

JOINT COMMISSION STANDARDS AND EMPLOYEE SAFETY

The Joint Commission addresses worker safety in several standards chapters. For example, the infection control standards address worker safety regarding infection control. However, the clearest statement of the Joint Commission's concern for employee safety occurs in the overview to the

SIDEBAR I-1. The Joint Commission's EC Management Plans

- Safety
- Security
- Hazardous Materials and Waste
- Emergency Management
- Fire Safety
- Medical Equipment
- Utilities

"Environment of Care" standards, which states, "The goal of this function is to provide a safe, functional, supportive and effective environment for patients, staff members, and other individuals in the organization." Included under this statement are all the safety, health, security, and violence-prevention concerns that could impact worker safety.

Within the context of their partnership, staff from the Joint Commission and OSHA identified examples of how health care organizations can comply with both OSHA regulations and Joint Commission standards without doing two different activities. Joint Commission and OSHA staff developed a cross-walk to validate common areas of compliance required of health care organizations. That cross-walk, updated to reflect the current standards, appears in Figure I-2, on page 4.

SURVEY/INSPECTION ACTIVITY

Although the Joint Commission surveyors and the OSHA inspectors are provided with education concerning the other agency's requirements, this is only intended to improve the efforts of both entities. Never in the history of the partnership has either organization inspected/surveyed for the other, nor is that the case now.

Joint Commission surveyors continue to survey a health care organization's performance against Joint Commission standards. However, surveyors are sensitive to how compliance meshes with OSHA expectations relative to the health and safety of the organization's employees. If deficiencies that relate to OSHA compliance are identified during an onsite survey, the surveyors will provide appropriate guidance and education materials as warranted.

CONTENT OF THE BOOK

Underscoring the renewal of the Joint Commission's partnership with OSHA, this book describes the intersection between the goals of these two organizations

INTRODUCTION

Figure I-1. Shared Strategies for a Safe and Healthy Work Environment[3]

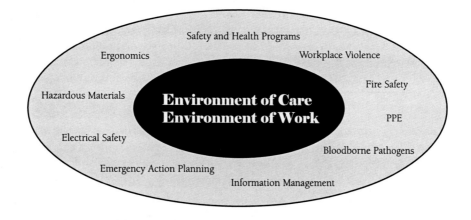

The Joint Commission's major concerns regarding health care workers and strategies for addressing them overlap concerns addressed in OSHA's regulations.

Source: *Environment of Care ® News,* December 2004, p. 2.

in promoting worker safety. Using Joint Commission standards and OSHA requirements as a foundation, the book breaks down worker safety issues into specific categories including facility, human factors, and clinically related risks, as well as performance measurement and improvement. Each chapter focuses on one of these categories and gives real-world examples of how to address worker safety issues that relate to these categories. The publication explores worker safety issues from an EC perspective and is designed to help health care organizations understand and focus on health care worker safety.

IMPORTANT DISTINCTIONS

Although this book references the OSHA requirements for worker safety, *the Joint Commission does **not** enforce compliance with OSHA standards.* OSHA requirements are provided here for consideration only, because they can help organizations to further ensure the safety of their workers. Please note that this book provides supplementary material to both the Joint Commission standards and the OSHA regulations. To be fully compliant with each organization's requirements, it is important to read the full text of the Joint Commission standards and the OSHA regulations.

FREQUENTLY USED TERMS

The Joint Commission defines the word *patient* as an individual who receives care treatment, and services, or one who may be represented by an appropriately authorized person. Within different types of health care organizations, a variety of synonyms for the word *patient* can include client, resident, and customer. In this book, to prevent confusion and ensure consistency, the term *patient* will be used universally to represent any individual served within a health care organization. ■

■ ■ ■ Figure I-2. Crosswalk of OSHA Topics to Joint Commission Standards [3]

OSHA Topic	Joint Commission Standards
BBP, TB, & Legionella	EC.1.10, Safety Management; EC.1.20, Security Management; EC.3.10, Hazardous Materials & Waste Management; EC.7.10, Utilities Management; EC.9.10, Monitoring Environmental Conditions; EC.9.20, Analyzing Environmental Issues; EC.9.30, Improving the Environment; HR.2.10, Initial Job Training; HR.2.20, Roles & Responsibilities; HR.2.30, Ongoing Education.
Confined Space	EC.1.10, Safety Management; HR.2.10, Initial Job Training; HR.2.20, Roles & Responsibilities; HR.2.30, Ongoing Education.
Education/Professional Qualifications of Parties Responsible for the Safety and Health Program	EC.1.10, Safety Management; HR.2.10, Initial Job Training; HR.2.20, Roles & Responsibilities; HR.2.30, Ongoing Education; LD.2.20, Effective Leadership.
Electrical Safety	EC.1.10, Safety Management; HR.2.10, Initial Job Training; HR.2.20, Roles & Responsibilities; HR.2.30, Ongoing Education.
Emergency Action Planning	EC.1.10, Safety Management; EC.4.10, Emergency Management; HR.2.10, Initial Job Training; HR.2.20, Roles & Responsibilities; HR.2.30, Ongoing Education.
ETO, H2CO, & Glutaraldehyde	EC.1.10, Safety Management; EC.1.20, Environmental Tours; EC.3.10, Hazardous Materials & Waste Management; EC.9.10, Monitoring Environmental Conditions; EC.9.20, Analyzing Environmental Issues; EC.9.30, Improving the Environment; HR.2.10, Initial Job Training; HR.2.20, Roles & Responsibilities; HR.2.30, Ongoing Education.
Fire Safety	EC.1.10, Safety Management; EC.5.10, Fire Safety; EC.5.20, LSC Compliance; EC.5.30, Fire Drills; EC.5.40, Fire Safety Equipment; EC.5.50, Interim Life Safety Measures; EC.9.10, Monitoring Environmental Conditions; EC.9.20, Analyzing Environmental Issues; EC.9.30, Improving the Environment; HR.2.10, Initial Job Training; HR.2.20, Roles & Responsibilities; HR.2.30, Ongoing Education.
Hazard Communication	EC.1.10, Safety Management; EC.3.10, Hazardous Materials & Waste Management; EC.9.10, Monitoring Environmental Conditions; HR.2.10, Initial Job Training; HR.2.20, Roles & Responsibilities; HR.2.30, Ongoing Education.
Information Management	IM.1.10, Planning & Design; IM.2.10, Information Privacy; IM.2.20, Information Security; IM.3.10, Information Management; IM.4.10, Decision Making; IM.5.10, Knowledge-Based Information; LD.4.50, Performance Improvement Priorities; LD.4.60, Resource Allocation; LD.4.70, Measuring Performance Improvement.
Laboratory and Hazcom	EC.1.10, Safety Management; EC.3.10, Hazardous Materials & Waste Management; EC.9.10, Monitoring Environmental Conditions; EC.9.20, Analyzing Environmental Issues; EC.9.30, Improving the Environment.
Machine Guarding	EC.1.10, Safety Management; HR.2.10, Initial Job Training; HR.2.20, Roles & Responsibilities; HR.2.30, Ongoing Education.
Patient Handling, Lifting, and Moving	EC.1.10, Safety Management; EC.9.10, Monitoring Environmental Conditions; EC.9.20, Analyzing Environmental Issues; EC.9.30, Improving the Environment; HR.2.10, Initial Job Training; HR.2.20, Roles & Responsibilities; HR.2.30, Ongoing Education.
Personal Protective Equipment	EC.1.10, Safety Management; EC.3.10, Hazardous Materials & Waste Management; EC.6.10, Medical Equipment Management; EC.7.10, Utilities Management; HR.2.10, Initial Job Training; HR.2.20, Roles & Responsibilities; HR.2.30, Ongoing Education.

continued

INTRODUCTION

Figure I-2. Crosswalk of OSHA Topics to Joint Commission Standards, continued

OSHA Topic	Joint Commission Standards
Safety & Health Programs	EC.1.10, Safety Management; EC.1.20, Environmental Tours; EC.9.10, Monitoring Environmental Conditions; EC.9.20, Analyzing Environmental Issues; EC.9.30, Improving the Environment; LD.3.80, Space, Equipment, & Resources.
Safety & Health Statistics, OSHA Record Keeping	EC.9.10, Monitoring Environmental Conditions; EC.9.20, Analyzing Environmental Issues; EC.9.30, Improving the Environment.
Ventilation	EC.1.20, Environmental Tours; EC.7.10, Utilities Management; EC.7.30, Utilities Maintenance; EC.7.50, Medical Gas & Vacuum; EC.8.10, Appropriate Environment; EC.8.30, Built Environment; EC.9.10, Monitoring Environmental Conditions; EC.9.20, Analyzing Environmental Issues.
Voluntary Protection Program	EC.1.10, Safety Management; EC.1.20, Environmental Tours; EC.2.10, Security Management; EC.3.10, Hazardous Materials & Waste Management; EC.8.10, Appropriate Environment; EC.9.10, Monitoring Environmental Conditions; EC.9.20, Analyzing Environmental Issues; EC.9.30, Improving the Environment.
Walking and Working Surfaces	EC.1.10, Safety Management; EC.1.20, Environmental Tours.
Workplace Violence	EC.1.10, Safety Management; EC.1.20, Environmental Tours; EC.2.10, Security Management; EC.9.10, Monitoring Environmental Conditions; EC.9.20, Analyzing Environmental Issues; EC.9.30, Improving the Environment

Many Joint Commission standards address topics similar to OSHA concerns.

References

1. Bureau of Labor Statistics, U.S. Department of Labor, Dec. 2002.

2. American Safety Training, Inc.: 29CFR *(Code of Federal Regulations) Part 1910 General Industry, 2nd ed.* Davenport, IA: American Safety Training, 2001.

3. Joint Commission: *The Environment of Care Series: OSHA and Environment of Care Compatibilities.* Oakbrook Terrace, IL: Joint Commission on Accreditation of Healthcare Organizations, 1998.

Chapter 1: OSHA Programs and Joint Commission Standards

Health care organizations are dedicated to the cure and healing of the ill and wounded. Simple consistency demands that they include within their mission the prevention of job-related illness and injury to their own workers. Both the Joint Commission and Occupational Safety and Health Administration (OSHA) support this concept through their own missions and requirements.

The crosswalk provided in the Introduction (pages 4–5) demonstrates the overlap between Joint Commission standards and OSHA requirements. This chapter will further explore that overlap by examining the following four OSHA programs and their support within the Joint Commission standards:

1. Safety and Health Programs
2. Voluntary Protection Programs
3. Hazard Communication
4. Recordkeeping and OSHA 300 Log

Safety and Health Programs

To ensure the safety of workers in an organization, leaders and their employees must be trained to recognize the hazards found in their environment and develop a comprehensive safety and health plan to prevent injuries and illnesses. Within their requirements, both the Joint Commission and OSHA emphasize the creation of this organizationwide safety plan. The Joint Commission requires organizations to assign someone or a team to coordinate the development, implementation, and monitoring of safety management activities. This individual is typically known as the *safety officer* (EC.1.10 and EC.9.10). The standards require organizations to conduct a proactive risk assessment and take a multidisciplinary approach to resolving safety issues. Policies and procedures are developed based on an organization's risk assessment process. Training programs must be implemented to inform new and current employees of their responsibilities to ensure their own safety, as well as the safety of the work environment.

STANDARDS *Joint Commission Standards that Address Safety*

➤ EC.1.10, Safety Management (EP4, EP6); EC.1.20, Environmental Tours; EC.3.10, Hazardous Materials & Waste Management; EC.4.20, Emergency Drills; EC.5.30, Fire Drills;

EC.5.40, Fire Safety Equipment; EC.6.20, Medical Equipment Maintenance; EC.7.30, Utilities Maintenance; EC.7.40, Emergency Power Systems; EC.7.50, Medical Gas & Vacuum; EC.9.10, Monitoring Environmental Conditions; EC.9.20, Analyzing Environmental Issues; EC.9.30, Improving the Environment
➤ LD.3.80, Space, Equipment, & Resources

Worker safety and health are directly linked to the existence and effectiveness of a safety and health program in a workplace.[1] In order to reduce employee injuries, health care organizations need to define, initiate, and maintain programs and procedures designed to prevent these injuries from occurring.

OSHA has standard elements that must be present in a safety and health program, and for that matter, any program involving OSHA compliance. Following are those elements:
- Management Leadership and Employee Participation
- Workplace Analysis
- Accident and Record Analysis
- Hazard Prevention and Control
- Safety and Health Training

Management Leadership

For a health care safety program to be effective, all employees, including physicians and volunteers, must be involved in the program. This involvement begins with keeping an open channel of communication between organization leaders, patients/residents/clients, visitors, and staff. Each management level must reflect an interest in safety and set a good example by complying with safety rules. Employees will believe in safety only to the degree to which they think their leaders believe in it. The leaders' interest in safety must be audible, visible, and continuous.[2] To be effective, leaders must do the following:
- Regularly communicate with staff about safety and health
- Provide staff with access to information relevant to the safety and health program
- Involve staff in hazard identification and assessment, hazard prioritization, instruction, and program evaluation
- Establish a way for staff to report hazards and injuries promptly and to make recommendations about appropriate ways to control these hazards
- Provide prompt responses to such reports and recommendations[3]

Leadership Support

Visible leadership provides the motivating force for an effective safety and health program. In fact, without it, the program is doomed to failure because an effective safety program must become part of an organization's culture.

It is essential that the leadership of a health care organization provides appropriate tools to the staff to implement a safety program. These tools would include the budget to support the program and staffing resources. Leadership must assign responsibility for the program to a qualified individual or team. Essentially, the health care organization itself has the discretion to determine the qualifications of this person or persons. For simplicity, this position will henceforth be referred to as the *safety officer*. In some large organizations, this may be a full-time position, filled by an individual with a degree in safety management. In other organizations, the safety officer may be one of many responsibilities borne by one person.

The Joint Commission requirements regarding the qualifications of a safety officer, as stated in EC.9.10, are as follows:
- Coordinates the ongoing organizationwide collection of information about deficiencies and opportunities for improvement in the environment of care
- Coordinates the ongoing collection and dissemination of other sources of information, such as published hazard notices or recall reports
- Coordinates the preparation of summaries of deficiencies, problems, failures, and user errors related to managing the environment of care
- Coordinates the preparation of summaries on findings, recommendations, actions taken, and results of performance improvement activities
- Participates in environmental tours and incident reporting
- Participates in developing safety policies and procedures

Note the frequent use of the words "coordinates" and "participates," further emphasizing the point that the safety officer is not the only person responsible for safety.

The theory of safety management suggests that the safety officer should report to senior management, such as to a vice presidential level or above. The reasons for this are twofold. First, reporting to senior management gives the safety officer both visibility and clout and lets the organization know that this position has the support of the administration. While managing the safety program, occasionally the safety officer must confront another employee over an issue of noncompliance or nonsupport. If the employee in question happens to be the safety officer's peer on the organizational chart, the confrontation has the potential to become difficult. Being able to access the vice president, for example, to intervene can be very helpful in the issue's resolution.

Second, if the safety officer must report through several layers of management to get to leadership, there is increased potential for interference with the process somewhere along the chain.

When designing a safety program, it is also important to have a process to review the program. Several opportunities for this are provided in Joint Commission standards. Perhaps the most obvious of these is found in EC.1.10 EP6, which states: "The organization establishes safety policies and procedures that are distributed, practiced, and reviewed as frequently as necessary, but at least every three years." It does not matter who reviews these documents; that is a matter of organizational policy. But a mechanism must be in place to conduct the review on schedule and to provide the associated documentation.

The standards also require a regular process of performance monitoring, which involves data collection and review to manage one or more aspects of each EC program. Based on this data, organizations can identify areas where they are struggling, or striving to improve. The data are reviewed and analyzed so that a performance improvement activity related to the environment of care can be recommended to the organization's leaders.

The standards also require organizations to conduct an annual evaluation of each environment of care program to assess its objectives, scope, performance, and effectiveness. This provides an annual opportunity to thoroughly review each of the seven environment of care management plans to determine where they succeed and where there are opportunities for improvement.

Employee Participation

Employee participation in the safety program provides a way that workers can identify hazards, recommend and monitor abatement, and otherwise participate in their own protection. OSHA calls for staff-level participation on an organization's safety committee. The Joint Commission requires representation on a multidisciplinary improvement team—often called the *safety* (or *environment of care*) *committee*—of clinical, administrative, and support services. Designation of representatives is solely at the discretion of the organization, and the size of the group should reflect the size and scope of the organization. Departments commonly considered for safety committee representation include the emergency department, employee health services, environmental services, facilities management, human resources, infection control, laboratory, medical staff, nursing, nursing support services, off-campus locations, radiology, risk management, and security.

TIP ▶ There are multiple ways to encourage employee participation in the safety program. Some organizations use a formal mechanism for any staff member to report a safety concern. This may take the form of a "safety hot line," where anyone can call to report an issue via a (frequently checked) recorded message. Another reporting venue is a "safety report form" process, whereby any staff member can fill out a form to submit a concern, either by name or anonymously. Obviously, it is important to promptly review all submissions, provide feedback when possible, and take action when necessary.

Another example of employee participation is the department safety liaison concept. Each department in the organization designates a safety liaison who is responsible for communicating safety information, ensuring safety training is complete, and essentially becoming the "champion" for safety in the department. Together the liaisons can form a safety team for the organization that provides two-way communication between the safety committee and the staff.

TIP ▶ Joint Commission's requirement for regular environmental tours, found in EC.1.20, provides another way to involve employees in safety efforts. Annual tours of the environment are required in all areas of a health care facility, and semiannually in areas where individuals are served. During these tours, it is common to ask questions of staff members in the area about their responsibilities in the environment of care regarding safety. Competition can be introduced between units for the "best score" on the tour, with awards or prizes given. This often promotes safety awareness and also staff enthusiasm for doing the right things the right way.

Workplace Analysis

An effective, proactive safety and health program will seek to identify and analyze all hazards. In large or complex workplaces, components of such analyses are the comprehensive survey and analysis of job hazards and changes in conditions. To identify new or previously missed hazards and failures in hazard controls, an effective safety and health program will include regular site inspections.

The environmental tours, mentioned on the previous page, are one mechanism for worksite analysis and risk assessment. The Joint Commission requires organizations to conduct environmental tours "to identify environmental deficiencies, hazards, and unsafe practices." Many organizations broaden this scope to address environment of care–related issues in addition to safety, such as assessment of *Life Safety Code*®* compliance, environmental cleanliness, infection control practice, nursing quality, and workers' compensation requirements. Results of these tours should be evaluated and reported, both to the safety committee and the department being toured. Documentation should be provided to "close the loop" and ensure that any issue is corrected.

The Joint Commission's standard EC.1.10 EP4 requires organizations to conduct comprehensive, proactive risk assessments that evaluate the potential adverse impact of buildings, grounds, equipment, occupants, and internal physical systems on the safety and health of patients, staff, and other people coming to the organization's facilities. Risk assessment is the ultimate goal of workplace analysis. It is a means by which the organization can manage the "gray areas" of safety – those for which there is no right or wrong answer. It requires continuous awareness of all processes and continuous questioning of their safety. Risk assessment issues should be brought to the safety committee, along with supporting information, where the issues are discussed and a conclusion reached regarding their management.

A reliable hazard reporting system, mentioned previously, enables employees, without fear of reprisal, to notify management of conditions that appear hazardous and to receive timely and appropriate responses. This is yet another component of worksite analysis and risk assessment.

Accident and Record Analysis

An effective safety program will provide for investigation of accidents and "near miss" incidents, so that their causes and the means for their prevention are identified. It is important to realize that actual accidents represent only the tip of the iceberg in terms of the magnitude of safety issues in organizations, and only by looking at near misses can a picture of the true magnitude of the problem come into view. Unfortunately, human nature is such that near misses and even actual occurrences frequently go unreported.

Accidents should be investigated as soon as possible after an event occurs to preserve the setting and memory of the individual involved. Investigations should be done objectively, with the intent of learning from the event, rather than punishing the individual involved. For example, an issue that arises in some accident investigations is worker fatigue. It stands to reason that workers will make more errors that can lead to accidents when they are tired. Getting enough rest is definitely a responsibility of the employee. However, the fiscal constraints of the organization with respect to staffing might also be examined if lack of sleep appears to be a recurring problem among employees.

An effective safety program will analyze injury and illness records (see "OSHA Recordkeeping and 300 Log," on page 21 of this chapter) for indications of sources and locations of hazards and jobs that experience higher numbers of injuries. Some OSHA standards, such as those relating to bloodborne pathogens, require an exposure control plan, whereby jobs are categorized as to their risk of exposure. Based on the

---

SIDEBAR 1-1. Contract Workers

When considering worker safety, do not neglect contract workers. An effective safety and health program protects all personnel on the worksite, including contractors. It is the responsibility of management to address contractor safety. In fact, during the on-site Joint Commission accreditation survey, the surveyors consider anyone who looks like he or she is doing work in the facility to be an "employee" of the organization, regardless of who signs his or her paycheck. This then includes various populations including agency nurses, independent practitioners, students, contract tradespeople, and service technicians.

The Joint Commission would expect these individuals to be familiar with their responsibilities in the environment of care regarding safety, as appropriate to their role and responsibilities in the health care organization. Because the Joint Commission considers all training to be role-specific, it is up to the organization to determine the appropriate EC training requirements for individuals in these positions, based on their job roles and the frequency of their presence in the facility.

Contractor training may be identical to new employee orientation, such as for an agency nurse, or it may be very different, such as a limited amount of printed information for a contract electrician who will be working in the building for one month.

---

* *Life Safety Code*® is a registered trademark of the National Fire Protection Association, Quincy, MA.

Chapter 1: OSHA Programs and Joint Commission Standards

exposure risk, employees are or are not recommended for hepatitis B vaccination. By analyzing injury and illness trends over time, patterns with common causes can be identified and prevented.

Hazard Prevention and Control

A key element of an organization's safety program is hazard prevention and control. Based on risks identified in a workplace analysis, organizations can implement controls to prevent or address any hazards. OSHA's requirements for hazard control involve a hierarchy of controls. Engineering controls are at the highest level of the hierarchy, and should be used whenever feasible to prevent or control hazards. These controls remove the hazard from a job or task by means of an engineered device or solution. Examples of engineering controls include a protected needle device used for phlebotomy work or a machine guard to prevent contact with a moving part.

The second level of controls, to be used if engineering controls are not feasible, is administrative or work practice controls. These represent the way individuals perform their work to reduce exposure to the hazard. When using this level of control, the hazard is still present, but is avoided by prudent practice and documented in policy or procedure. Examples of this type of control include prohibitions of unsafe practices such as prohibiting the use of the top rung of a ladder or the recapping of needles. Another would be limiting the exposure of workers to a hazard by limiting the time or frequency of exposure. An example of this would be limiting the time any individual could wear level B personal protective equipment (PPE) in a decontamination procedure without a rest period to avoid the heat hazard.[4]

Finally, the lowest level of the hierarchy of hazard control is PPE . PPE is provided to the worker to individually protect him or her from a hazard that cannot be removed from the environment and/or limited in exposure. Numerous examples of PPE are used in health care, including gloves, safety goggles, protective aprons, respiratory protection, and many others. (During a Joint Commission accreditation survey, use of personal protective equipment is usually addressed under EC.3.10, Hazardous Materials & Waste.) More about PPE can be found in Chapter Three.

Equipment Maintenance

An effective safety and health program will provide for facility and equipment maintenance to prevent hazardous breakdowns. There are many requirements throughout the "Environment of Care" chapter of the accreditation manuals relating to inspecting, testing, and maintaining equipment. These functions are clearly required for features of fire protection in EC.5.40, for medical equipment in EC.6.20, for utilities systems in EC.7.30, and in particular for emergency power supply systems in EC.7.40 and medical gas in EC.7.50. To look at it more broadly, the environmental tours represent inspecting, testing, and maintaining a safe environment. The scoring algorithms for these standards set clear expectations, depending on the criticality of the equipment or component, for preventive maintenance completion rates. For example, the most critical medical equipment providing life support must have a preventive maintenance completion rate of 100%.

Emergency Response

Both the Joint Commission's and OSHA's requirements regarding a health and safety program mandate appropriate planning, training, and drills for emergency response, along with the provision of appropriate equipment. For example, the Joint Commission expects fire drills to be conducted once per shift per quarter in health care occupancies and once per shift per year in business occupancies. All employees on all shifts must participate to the extent called for in the organization's fire plan.

Emergency drills should be conducted twice a year, at least four months but no more than eight months apart in health care occupancies. Business occupancies must conduct at least one emergency drill annually. Organizations that are designated to receive victims in a communitywide emergency must include one drill with an influx of volunteer or simulated patients. And, where applicable, these organizations must also participate in a communitywide drill.

Safety and Health Training

According to the Joint Commission and OSHA, safety and health training should cover the safety and health responsibilities of all personnel who work at the site or affect the operations. OSHA regulations state that training is required for all employees who may be at risk from the hazards in their work areas. This includes all employees, regardless of hiring status (permanent, part-time, or temporary), as well as contract/ agency employees and volunteers. The training must be completed before an employee is put at risk for exposure.[5] Additional training would be required any time a new hazard is introduced, and refresher training must be provided periodically. The Joint Commission's human resources chapter of each program's accreditation manual contains standards requiring initial orientation and training, ongoing education and training, and job-specific duties or responsibilities relative to safety.

Supervisors should be trained to analyze the work under their supervision, maintain physical protection of their work areas, reinforce employee training, and enforce organization safety policies, as necessary. Organization leaders are responsible for ensuring that all training is provided by qualified individuals. Several OSHA requirements address the issue of safety training. A summary of these is provided in Figure 1-1 on page 13.

While the previous sections discuss the myriad components necessary for an effective safety and health program, the case study below illustrates how all the components of a safety and health program come together to improve the safety of workers and patients.

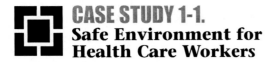

CASE STUDY 1-1.
Safe Environment for Health Care Workers

Matrix Helps Carolinas HealthCare System Keep Close Watch

When the number of employee ergonomic injuries at Sardis Oaks Nursing Home dropped significantly in three years, Carolinas HealthCare System (CHS) administrators knew their initiative begun in 2000 to secure safer environments for patients, visitors, and personnel was paying off. That was the objective, according to CHS's Director of Safety Diana Ash, that set in motion their laudable and innovative approach to safety management.

Carolinas HealthCare System is a diverse, not-for-profit network of owned, leased, and managed operations serving both North and South Carolina. With more than 4,300 licensed beds and 25,300 employees, it is "the largest healthcare system in the Carolinas, and the fourth largest public system in the nation." CHS has developed an environmental, health, and safety program that supports a culture of safety where communications are streamlined and issues are proactively examined and addressed.

Using a Matrix to Identify Areas for Improvement

One of the important components of CHS's program is its comprehensive Regulatory Assessment Matrix for organizational self-rating. This matrix breaks out several categories of the Joint Commission's Environment of Care (EC) safety standards and identifies their corresponding regulatory agencies, including the Occupational Safety and Health Administration (OSHA), the Environmental Protection Association (EPA), the National Fire Protection Association (NFPA), and so forth. The matrix also includes CHS's own programs, policies and practices regarding the environment of care and safety. (See Figure 1-2.)

The Regulatory Matrix color-codes the status of any designated program area in green, yellow, or red to indicate full, partial, or noncompliance, respectively. This comprehensive grid allows the safety officer for each CHS facility to readily identify areas that are in compliance as well as those needing attention. Safety officers can also use the matrix to spot, at a glance, any overlapping compliance areas. For example, CHS, the Joint Commission, OSHA, and NFPA all mandate some programs or activities concerning fire safety and personal protective equipment, including eye, face, foot, hand, and head protection. These regulations are identified by appropriate number(s) in their corresponding columns to the right of the descriptive fields for each program area.

The matrix not only improves CHS's overall safety monitoring, but "it offers many economies of scale. It helps avoid duplication of effort and thus increases efficiency in compliance activities for the individual facilities," claimed Ash. For example, safety officers who are required to conduct regularly scheduled annual or biannual safety tours of their facilities can easily monitor several agencies' requirements simultaneously using the matrix. In addition, the matrix tool may be used to facilitate reporting to agencies: "One column on the Regulatory Matrix is devoted to Joint Commission issues. But we have also developed a Joint Commission scoring worksheet that supplements the matrix. The worksheet allows us to further prepare for accreditation activities," explained Marsha Wallace, CHS safety analyst, who also ensures compliance with

Chapter 1: OSHA Programs and Joint Commission Standards

Figure 1-1. OSHA Training Requirements for Health Care Facilities[6]

Topic	Description	Frequency of Training
Personal Protective Equipment	Required for any employee required to wear personal protective equipment, such as latex gloves or a respirator	Upon assignment and annually thereafter, with refresher training required for a job change or introduction of new equipment or processes
Confined Spaces	Required for all employees whose work is subject to a confined space (such as in a manhole or crawl space)	Upon assignment and annually thereafter
Hazard Communication	Required for anyone who works in an area containing hazardous chemicals	Upon assignment and annually thereafter, with refresher training required for a job change or introduction of new equipment or processes
Fire Extinguishers	Required for anyone expected to use a fire extinguisher	Upon assignment and annually thereafter
Emergency Action	All employees must be trained in the emergency procedures of the facility (for example, fire and evacuation).	Upon assignment and annually thereafter
Bloodborne Pathogens	Required for all employees for whom occupational exposure may take place	Upon assignment and annually thereafter
Machine Guarding	Required for all employees who work in maintenance shops or around electric mixers, meat slicers, and so on	Upon assignment, with refresher training required for a job change or introduction of new equipment or processes
Workplace Violence	Recommended to enable employees to react to violence inflicted by patients, fellow employees, or outsiders	Upon assignment and annually thereafter

Here is a summary of OSHA requirements addressing safety training.
Source: *Environment of Care® News,* May/June 2001, p. 6–7.

OSHA and other agencies. One further benefit of the matrix is its applicability to the many different types of facilities in the CHS system, from a teaching hospital to nursing homes to outpatient facilities, obviating the need for individualized assessment tools.

Applying Results Across the System

After each facility's safety officer uses the matrix to generate a report on safety, the CHS Corporate Safety department evaluates these reports to identify the whole system's strengths and areas for improvement. This annual Strength/Witness/Opportunity/Threat Analysis (SWOT) provides the corporate safety department with information to use in developing their annual action plans. "The Regulatory Matrix gives us an overview—the pulse—of the system," explained Ash. "We prioritize any red areas and monitor the yellow and green. We can't work on everything at once, so we target 5-10 areas each year for improvement." The printout of the SWOT Analysis displays a numeric score, indicating the compliance level of each area targeted for focus. It also uses a color-coded "dashboard rating" system, which, like the matrix design, enables parties to immediately visualize progress and compliance in multiple focus areas.

CHS Corporate Safety department reviews and summarizes the cumulative matrix data annually and develops a Safety and Environmental Action Plan (SEAP) with the

CHS corporate compliance department and the facility safety officers, focusing on those areas to be targeted for the coming year. At the corporate level, the safety department staff creates a Tactical Program Goal(s) Summary to support the facility safety officers in the implementation of their plans. One tactical goal set for 2005 is the development and installation of a centralized, online reporting program for tracking employee incidents, which will enable the facility's safety officers and safety committees, as well as department managers, to initiate preventive measures. "We are looking to see if there is a correlation in incidents across facilities to identify and eliminate problem areas," explained Ash.

Following the review and tactical goals summary the safety programs are implemented. This process includes establishing performance measures. Implementing the programs in the facilities requires identifying the appropriate, specialized staff who can expedite the goals of the program, including experts in lab safety, hazardous materials, and other critical areas as well as CHS EC Committee members and the facility safety officers.

Using Education to Ensure Safety

Another notable component in the CHS safety program is the proprietary employee training or Annual Continuing Education (ACE) modules. Like the Regulatory Matrix Assessment, employee training is an evolving feature of CHS's safety program that has expanded greatly from its original inception. The CHS Corporate Safety department, along with support from CHS Employee Development, creates and maintains numerous online training modules for employees throughout the system. In addition to the required core modules, all employees must view units that are specific to their departments and/or disciplines. Employees have a specified timeline for completion of viewing their respective modules, are tested annually, and must receive a minimum passing grade of 85%. Employees are allowed up to three tries to pass each module.

Employees are trained and tested on a wide range of topics concerning their own safety, including, but not limited to, the following:
- General environment of care
- Ergonomics
- Bloodborne pathogens
- Personal protective equipment
- Radiation safety for dental and radiology personnel
- Fire safety in a health care setting
- General safety
- Safe use of hazardous materials
- Emergency management
- Airborne precautions
- Portable liquid oxygen
- Respiratory protection
- Hazard communication
- Medical equipment management
- Utilities management

Employees are also trained on other issues such as patient safety, government policies, and facility security.

In addition to their mandatory annual module testing, 5% of employees are randomly tested by the facility's Employee Health Department as part of a safety checkup test program. This helps determine how well employees have retained the information in the modules. This random testing is performed in conjunction with the random drug testing program. Ash views this method as a good way to measure staff education. For example, a short random test may consist of 8-10 questions tied to the employees' general knowledge of such safety areas as hazardous materials, life safety, emergency management, and fire or electrical safety. Based on the random testing results, modules may be updated or added, as necessary, to reinforce the employees' information retention and performance. "We want to make sure that employees remember information and can apply it to circumstances out on the floor," said Ash.

Commitment to Culture of Safety

The final critical component in the CHS safety program is corporate management's support of and commitment to the culture of safety, which Ash feels is vital to CHS's success. This is mandated by senior management in the CHS Corporate Environmental, Health, and Safety Business Plan. One way this is accomplished is through an allotted corporate department budget of more than $1 million to recruit the necessary personnel; develop and maintain

Chapter 1: OSHA Programs and Joint Commission Standards

Figure 1-2. Carolinas HealthCare System Environment, Health, and Safety Regultory Matrix Assessment Tool

Dashboard Rating -	Program Design for the Environment of Care (EOC)	CHS Policies/Tools/Programs/Best Practice	JCAHO	OSHA	EPA	NFPA	DOT	WC/EH Risk Mgmt
	Choose Color Code: Please self-rate your preparation/compliance activities for each item. For items which do not apply choose a Blue to indicate NA. The absence of a program/required compliance activities = RED, partial compliance = YELLOW and compliance = GREEN							
	EDUCATION							
	Orientation (*Initial*)							
	New Manager/Director Orientation	Safety Mgmt Plan, Corporate Compliance Policies	EC.1.20					
	New Employee Orientation	Safety Mgmt Plan, Corporate Compliance Policies	EC.1.20					
	Responsibilities and Authority of the Safety Committee/Chairperson	CHS 1.01	EC.1.20					
	Responsibilities and Authority of Managers and Directors	CHS 1.02	EC.1.20					
	Functions of Facility Safety Officer	FSO Job Description	EC.1.20					
	Enforcement of Safety Rules and Regulations	CHS1.03	EC.1.20					
	ACE Modules (*Annual*): ALL EMPLOYEES - Mandatory	CHS 1.07						
	General Safety (EOC)	CHS-SMPM Section 2	EC.1.10, EC.1.20					
	Security in the Healthcare Setting	CHS 2.08, CHS-SMPM Section 10	EC.2.10					
	Safe Medical Device Act	CHS 3.07, CHS 3.08	EC.6.10					
	Medical Equipment Management and Utilities Management	CHS 3.04, CHS 10.02(a), 10.02(l), 10.02(m), 10.02(n)	E6.20 EC.7.10					
	Emergency Management	CHS - SMPM Section 10	EC.4.10	29CFR 1910.38, 29CFR 1910.119, 29CFR 1910.120, 29CFR 1910.165, 29CFR 1910.1200				
	Performance Improvement		EC.9.10 EC.9.20 EC.9.30					
	Bloodborne Pathogens	CHS 7.01	EC.1.10, EC.1.20	29CFR 1910.1030				
	Infection Control	CHS 7.05	EC.1.10, EC.1.20					
	Infant Abduction	CHS 10.02(f) Code Pink	EC.2.10					x
	Corporate Compliance							
	Personal Protective Equipment		EC.1.10, EC.1.20	29CFR 1910.132, 29CFR 1910.133, 29CFR 1910.134, 29CFR 1910.135, 29CFR 1910.136, 29CFR 1910.137, 29CFR 1910.138, 29CFR 1910.139				
	Fire Safety	CHS - SMPM Section 4	EC.5.10	29CFR 1910.38, 29CFR 1910.157				
	Hazard Communication	CHS - SMPM Section 6	EC.3.10	29CFR 1910.1200				

A sample page from Carolinas HealthCare System's Matrix.

Source: Carolina's HealthCare System.

---

appropriate tools, training programs, and policies; implement corporate programs; and comply with all applicable regulatory standards.

CHS is one of few systems whose safety program ties into OSHA's Voluntary Protection Program, resulting in numerous benefits including, according to Ash, "reduced injury rates and lost work days due to injuries, improved working conditions, decreased treatment costs, increased production, improved employee morale, and enhanced labor-management relationships."

Better safety management at CHS is an ongoing objective that can never be perfect yet is always improving. With the utilization of the Regulatory Matrix and the ACE modules, CHS is committed to setting and achieving the highest safety standards at all their facilities, thus establishing and maintaining a safe workplace.

Case at a Glance

Main Challenge: To improve employee safety and reduce safety incidents

Issues: To comply with regulatory drivers; to educate staff; to ensure corporate backing of a "culture of safety" EC Standards: **EC.1.10** and **EP 5**

Solutions: Developed an innovative color-coded tracking and trending matrix to graphically monitor compliance in employee safety; created online education modules for employees and monitor success of education efforts via annual and random spot testing for employee knowledge; implement systemwide strategies and plans based on program feedback.

Outcomes: By developing several innovative programs, creating strategic plans based on data summaries and analysis, and fostering an integrated approach between management and facilities personnel to implement safety plans, CHS realized a significant decrease in employee safety incidents at the field level.[7]

Voluntary Protection Programs

Any organization having an exemplary safety and health program could consider applying for acceptance into OSHA's Voluntary Protection Programs (VPP). The program emphasizes the importance of worksite safety and health programs in meeting the goal of the Occupational Safety and Health Act. The VPP is voluntary, as the name implies, and provides public recognition for the organization as well as removal from programmed OSHA inspection lists. The health care organization further benefits from VPP status in that it should expect to see increased quality and productivity due to the increased motivation for safety. The organization should also see fewer lost workdays and therefore decreased workers' compensation costs.

Under the VPP, OSHA recognizes that the organization far exceeds the basic elements of ongoing systematic protection of workers at the site. Therefore, these sites do not need routine federal enforcement activities. The VPP sites are also used as resources and examples by OSHA, and provide input into the standard setting process.

After an organization has submitted its VPP application, OSHA will conduct an on-site visit to verify the contents of the application. This program review will be conducted by a team, which includes at least a team leader, a safety specialist, and an industrial hygienist. The review typically lasts about four days. The organization must commit to correcting any OSHA deficiencies discovered during this review, but no enforcement action will be taken.[8]

Application for participation in the VPP program should not be taken lightly. The Joint Commission standards provide a framework that is compatible with the OSHA VPP process, but Joint Commission compliance is not sufficient for VPP participation. The VPP requires a significant amount of documentation and commitment from the organization. If a health care organization knows that it has an exemplary safety and health program and is willing to make the commitment, application to the OSHA VPP should be considered. Additional information may be found at www.osha.gov/dcsp/vpp. As of July 30, 2004, there were 17 health services organizations participating in the federal OSHA VPP.

The following case study[9] illustrates how one hospital successfully met the VPP requirements.

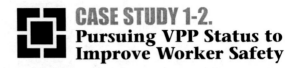

CASE STUDY 1-2.
Pursuing VPP Status to Improve Worker Safety

Blake Medical Center Achieves Star Status

Blake Medical Center, a full-service acute care hospital located in Bradenton, Florida, had a history of many successful Joint Commission surveys. To build on that culture of quality and safety, it invited inspectors from the Occupational Safety and Health Administration (OSHA) to its door.

In January 2000, Blake began seeking membership in OSHA's elite Voluntary Protection Program (VPP). The VPP allows participants with comprehensive safety and health programs to be removed from OSHA's regular inspection lists and avoid fines during scheduled OSHA inspections. Being part of the VPP also helps Blake meet Joint Commission requirements. "That OSHA partnered with the Joint Commission was one of the positive reasons to get into the VPP," said Andre Scharroo, Blake's director of environmental services. "The alliance means more emphasis on a safe workforce and safe patient, and it creates an overall culture of safety in the hospital."

"Membership in the Voluntary Protection Program also shows employees that our organization is committed to a safe working environment. This can improve staff morale and performance," stated Brenda Wehrle, vice president of quality/risk for Blake Medical Center.

Working Toward the Goal

The first step to achieving membership in VPP was to have unequivocal management support. Blake set a goal to achieve VPP star status. This goal was included in the organization's strategic plan, thus emphasizing leadership's commitment to the process. "The strategic plan sets specific goals and objectives for the organization as a whole, as well as for each department and employee. By including VPP star status as a goal in our strategic plan, we were able to drive the organization's efforts to achieve the goal," stated Wehrle.

Chapter 1: OSHA Programs and Joint Commission Standards

To prepare for OSHA's arrival, Blake examined the six elements of the VPP program:
1. Management leadership and employee participation
2. Job hazard/workplace hazard analysis
3. Accident and record analysis
4. Hazard prevention and control
5. Emergency response and emergency preparedness
6. Safety and health training

"Each element has specific requirements that organizations must meet in order to receive VPP merit status. To receive VPP star status, organizations must exceed these requirements," stated Wehrle. Blake compared the requirements for each element with the components of its safety and health program, and made modifications where improvement was necessary.

Blake submitted its application to OSHA. It was reviewed and received VPP merit status for meeting OSHA's requirements. "While we were pleased, we weren't satisfied with merit status; our goal was to achieve star status," stated Dorothy Lenz, employee/occupational health nurse for Blake Medical Center.

Building on Success

To achieve star status, the organization further refined its safety and health program. One area where the organization made improvements was in job hazard analysis. Historically, Blake had conducted an overall assessment of risk to determine job hazards. OSHA required that the organization do a job hazard analysis for each task in the organization. "The OSHA surveyor showed us a way to effectively conduct a job hazard analysis and we adopted that format," said Lenz. "It is an easy-to-use format that involves the employee in the analysis process. It allows us to analyze job hazards and also train employees on job hazards at the same time."

Blake also improved its handling of hazardous materials. The organization had already changed its spill procedures so that every department was trained to clean up its own spills. To achieve star status, the organization worked to reduce the use of hazardous chemicals in the organization. "We eliminated the use of ethylene oxide (EtO) in the facility, thus improving both worker and patient safety. When we do need to purchase chemicals, such as formaldehyde, we buy them in small containers only, to reduce the scope of potential spills," stated Lenz.

Blake also worked to eliminate the presence of mercury in the organization. "We are almost mercury free. We have two mercury thermometers that are needed for equipment found in the lab. Other than those two thermometers, the organization has eliminated the use of mercury in the facility," said Lenz.

By striving to achieve VPP star status, Blake Medical Center was also able to better meet Joint Commission standards. For instance, the hospital found that it could reduce staff injuries—back strains, slips, and falls—when moving patients from beds to stretchers. By using an inflatable patient transfer safety device, the organization not only improved worker safety, but greatly increased patient safety and security. The device is an inflatable piece of soft, parachute-like nylon on which the patient is positioned. After the device is

---

Case at a Glance

Main Challenge: Achieve OSHA's Voluntary Protection Program star status to help improve patient and staff safety throughout the organization. Star status also helps reduce the number of onsite visits from OSHA, decrease workers' compensation costs, and can improve staff morale.

Issues: VPP star status requires an organization to exceed the requirements set down by OSHA regarding worker safety. Although organizations can use Joint Commission standards to prepare for the VPP survey, OSHA's requirements for VPP membership go beyond those outlined by the Joint Commission.

Joint Commission Standards: EC.1.10, EC.1.20, EC.3.10, EC.4.10, EC.8.10, EC.9.10, EC.9.20, EC.9.30

Solutions: Blake compared its safety program to OSHA's requirements and implemented initiatives to improve safety where necessary. For example, the organization conducted improvement initiatives in the areas of job hazard analysis, patient safety, and hazardous materials and waste.

Outcomes: The organization first received VPP merit status, which indicated that OSHA's requirements were met. A year and a half later, the organization received VPP star status, showing that the organization exceeded OSHA's requirements.

plugged in it inflates, hugs, and supports the patient. The device allows two people to move a large patient very easily and safely from a bed to a stretcher without straining themselves or hurting the patient. The device even allows an x-ray to pass through it.

In addition to this device, the organization created the Safe Handling of Patients (SHOP) team that was charged with examining additional patient safety equipment. "Increased patient safety can translate into increased worker safety," stated Lenz. "By looking for equipment that helped improve patient safety, we were addressing the needs of employees also."

Achieving the Goal

Eighteen months after OSHA awarded Blake with VPP merit status, Blake invited OSHA inspectors to return to the organization. Upon surveying Blake's safety program again, OSHA awarded the organization with VPP star status.

VPP membership has had several benefits. It has helped Blake meet its Joint Commission requirements and reduced workers' compensation costs. In addition, management has noticed improved employee motivation to work safely, and the organization has received high-profile kudos. "We received a letter from Governor Jeb Bush recognizing us," said Wehrle.

Although surprise visits from OSHA are a thing of the past, OSHA will continue to inspect Blake. "We have to conduct an annual assessment of our safety program and submit a report to OSHA," stated Wehrle. "OSHA will also come onsite periodically to make sure we still meet the requirements of the VPP." It has been three years since Blake received its star status, and the organization is preparing for a follow-up visit from OSHA. Provided this visit is successful, OSHA will visit onsite and conduct a follow-up inspection every five years.

In addition to OSHA, Blake regularly monitors the effectiveness of the safety and health program. "We monitor injury rates throughout the organization to see if we need to implement initiatives to reduce these rates, such as increased training and education for staff," stated Lenz.

"Achieving VPP status is hard work, but it is worth it," Wehrle noted. "We take great pride in our history of success with the Joint Commission. And this is another level of success."

HAZARD COMMUNICATION (HAZCOM)

Both the Joint Commission and OSHA address the risks associated with hazardous materials and waste. Joint Commission standard EC.3.10 requires organizations to manage their hazardous materials and waste risks. EP1 requires organizations to create a written management plan describing how hazardous materials and waste are managed. OSHA's Hazard Communication Standard is 29CFR 1910.1200. This standard is considered one of the "right to know" laws, stating that an employee has the right to know about hazardous chemicals in use in the workplace.

STANDARDS *Joint Commission Standards that Address Hazardous Materials and Waste*

➤ EC.1.10, Safety Management; EC.3.10 Hazardous Materials & Waste Management (EP1, EP2, EP9, EP12), EC.9.10, Monitoring Environmental Conditions
➤ HR.2.10, Initial Job Training; HR.2.20, Roles & Responsibilities; HR.2.30, Ongoing Education

OSHA has specific requirements for topics to be included in an organization's hazard communication plan:
1. Hazard Communication Program: Introduction to the process and statement of purpose for the program; includes information about hazard determination
2. Chemical Inventory: Statement of how this process occurs and what to do for discrepancies
3. Material Safety Data Sheets (MSDS): Explanation of MSDS and how to obtain them within the organization
4. Labels and Other Forms of Warning: Labeling requirements and expectations for use
5. Hazardous Nonroutine Tasks: Definition of these tasks, and explanation of training
6. Employee Training and Information: Details later in this chapter

Chapter 1: OSHA Programs and Joint Commission Standards

Hazard Determination

Chemical manufacturers and importers are responsible for evaluating their chemicals to determine if they are hazardous. Health care (and other) employers do not have to perform a separate evaluation and can choose to rely on the manufacturers' or importers' determination. According to OSHA, this is a performance-oriented process, with no specifically prescribed methods. It relies heavily on professional judgment, but a scientifically defensible determination must be made. Chemical manufacturers must evaluate their products based on carcinogenicity, human data, animal data, and the adequacy of reporting data. After a material is determined to be hazardous under this standard, requirements are put in place for an annual chemical inventory, staff education, material safety data sheets (MSDS), and labeling of the chemicals.

Many chemicals found within health care organizations are also found in typical households, such as bleach. The requirements for an MSDS are based on the use of the chemical. For example, if an environmental services employee put a small amount of bleach into each of four loads of laundry during the day, that would be considered normal household use and an MSDS would not be required. If another employee was assigned to clean restrooms using bleach all day every day, this would be in excess of normal household use, and an MSDS would be required.

Inventory of Hazardous Chemicals

EP2 of EC.3.10 requires organizations to make an inventory of hazardous materials stored, used, or generated using "criteria consistent with applicable law and regulation." OSHA provides one source of that law and regulation. OSHA also requires an annual inventory of the chemicals used within a facility. This is a difficult undertaking, but one that must be accomplished to be in compliance with both organizations. After an initial physical inventory has been taken, it is easier to keep the inventory updated on an annual basis. It is helpful to have some inventory control on chemicals being ordered and to enforce a policy that all chemicals must come through materials management (as opposed to buying them at the local hardware store).

Per OSHA's requirements, each of the chemicals on the inventory list must have an available MSDS. The MSDS contains information in English provided by the chemical manufacturer including the chemical name and manufacturer, hazardous ingredients and associated exposure limits, physical properties, fire and explosion information, health hazards, toxicology information, reactivity and incompatibility, spill response, special protection required, and storage and handling[4].

MSDS must be available to the employees in the organization in their work area during their work shift. This does not necessarily mean that each department must have a file of paper MSDS for the chemicals in use, although that certainly is acceptable. Both Joint Commission and OSHA will accept electronic MSDS. No matter what format the MSDS take, it is important that every employee be able to access them.

Note that for exposure limits, OSHA uses "Permissible Exposure Limits" or PELs. These are OSHA's legally allowed concentration of airborne contaminants in the workplace, and are of three types:

- 8-hour Time Weighted Average (TWA): The employee's average airborne exposure in any 8-hour work shift in a 40-hour work week, which shall not be exceeded.
- Short-Term Exposure Limit (STEL): The employee's 15 minute time-weighted average exposure that shall not be exceeded at any time in a work day unless another time period is specified.
- Ceiling: The employee's exposure that shall not be exceeded during any part of the work day.

These limits are derived from the American Conference of Government Industrial Hygienists (ACGIH) Threshold Limit Values (TLVs). TLVs are airborne concentrations of substances and represent conditions under which nearly all workers may be repeatedly exposed on a daily basis without adverse effect. TLVs are not mandatory federal or state exposure standards.

Labeling

Chemical labeling is another aspect of the Hazard Communication Standard, and it is also reflected in EC.3.10 EP12, "The organization properly labels hazardous materials and waste." According to OSHA, all chemical labels must contain, at a minimum, the identity of the chemical, the name and contact information of the manufacturer, and any hazard information about the chemical.

If chemicals are placed in secondary containers, these must also be labeled as above, with the exception of a container used by one employee on one work shift. In other words, if a laboratory technologist poured a small amount of methanol from a large bottle to be used at his or her work station during the day and discarded it at the end of the shift, the smaller container would be acceptable without a label. If that same small container was shared by several technologists or used over several shifts, it would require an appropriate label.

Hazardous Nonroutine Tasks

Some employees are occasionally asked to perform tasks outside their normal routine. For example, an environmental services employee could occasionally be asked to clean the laboratory in place of a fellow worker who was on vacation. In this case, the substitute employee would need to be briefed about the hazardous chemicals stored and used in the laboratory prior to filling the assignment.

Employee Training

Both the Joint Commission and OSHA emphasize the importance of training employees about the risks associated with hazardous materials and waste. Joint Commission's HR and EC standards both address the issue. For example, EC.3.10 EP9 requires appropriate procedures and PPE to be available for hazardous materials and waste spills or exposures. HR.2.20 requires all staff to be able to describe or demonstrate their roles and responsibilities relative to safety. See the case study on page 16.

Orientation and training is required by OSHA under the Hazard Communication Standard. All employees must be trained to know the requirements of the standard, and the following:
- The presence of hazardous chemicals in their work area
- The location and availability of the Hazard Communication plan
- The location and availability of the chemical inventory and MSDS
- Detection of the presence or accidental release of hazardous chemicals
- The physical and health hazards of chemicals in their work area
- Ways to protect themselves from the hazards
- Details of the organization's Hazard Communication Program
- Procedures for an emergency spill or exposure[10]

Additional training is required any time a new chemical is introduced into the workplace, there is a change in formulation of a chemical already in use, or new hazard information becomes available about an existing chemical.

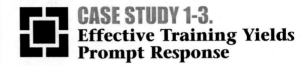

CASE STUDY 1-3.
Effective Training Yields Prompt Response

Mercury Cleanup in an Ambulatory Care Organization

Due to the nature or their work, health care organizations can be vulnerable to chemical and other hazardous materials spills. The ramifications of a spill can be expensive, time-consuming, and harmful to patients, staff, and visitors. Quick response to a spill can prevent injury as well as minimize costs.

Circle Family Care, Inc., a nonprofit ambulatory organization located on Chicago's West Side, discovered an accidental mercury spill in one of its clinic's exam rooms. A mercury-containing sphygmomanometer was dislodged from the wall and fell to the floor. The equipment broke on impact and caused mercury to spill in the room.

Inhaled mercury is harmful to humans, with children being more susceptible to mercury poisoning than adults. Even brief contact with low levels of mercury can have damaging health effects, including loss of appetite, fatigue, insomnia, and changes in behavior or personality. Mercury vapors can be breathed in and are readily absorbed by the lungs.

Circle Family Care provides community health services, behavioral health services, and children and family support services. Clients range in age from newborn to geriatric and thus the effects of a mercury spill could be devastating. It was important that Circle Family Care immediately address the mercury spill in a way that would minimize the health risks for their staff, clients, and visitors.

The spill was discovered when a provider and a client entered the room for an exam. After the spill was found, the provider did not allow the client to enter further into the room and immediately closed off the area. A nurse then entered the room wearing proper PPE and, using the proper precautionary techniques, applied an internal spill kit to the area.

Circle Family Care has a specific policy and procedure that outline the proper precautionary techniques, PPE and other equipment needed, and actions that should follow a chemical spill such as this one. "The nurse knew what to do because all organizational staff are required to attend annual safety training as part of our overall training and education program. The policy and procedure relating to mercury spill cleanup are part of that training," said Michael Patterson, operations supervisor at Circle Family Care.

In addition to applying the initial spill kit, Circle Family Care called the fire department, and the fire department's chemical spill unit handled the secondary cleanup process.

Because staff acted quickly and immediately closed off the exam room, the mercury was not tracked to any other part of the facility and no additional areas of the facility needed to be closed. There was no impact to clients, staff, or visitors because the room was closed immediately before mercury contamination could spread. By having the staff thoroughly trained on response procedures, Circle Family Care was able to respond quickly and appropriately to the situation.

Circle Family Care was fortunate that the nature of the spill was limited and immediate containment was possible. However, the organization did not want to count on such luck again. To prevent this type of event from happening in the future, Circle Family Care has identified, throughout its facility, similar units to the one that broke. Within six months, these units were replaced by new equipment that does not contain mercury. "Although it is expensive, replacing all the equipment will be cheaper than the consequences of having another unit fall," said Patterson.[11]

Contractor Information

Contractors must be provided with information about the hazardous materials used and/or stored in the areas of the facility in which they are working. OSHA requirements for this are similar to those for organizational employees. Conversely, contractors must also inform the organization of any hazardous materials that they bring to the worksite and provide appropriate MSDS.

OSHA RECORDKEEPING AND 300 LOG

To help track worker safety in an organization, organizations should document staff illness and injuries. Although the Joint Commission requires this, OSHA's requirements are much more prescriptive on this issue. OSHA requires all employers with 11 or more employees to keep injury and illness records on the OSHA 300 Log, which is a log and summary of occupational illnesses. In addition employers must file an incident report of occupational illnesses and injuries on a separate form.

STANDARDS *Joint Commission Standards that Address Recordkeeping*

➤ EC.9.10, Monitoring Environmental Conditions; EC.9.20, Analyzing Environmental Issues; EC.9.30, Improving the Environment

OSHA defines an occupational illness as "any abnormal condition or disorder, other than one resulting from an occupational injury, caused by exposure to environmental factors associated with employment. It includes acute and chronic illnesses or diseases that may be caused by inhalation, absorption, ingestion, or direct contact." These would include skin diseases, such as contact dermatitis, and repetitive trauma disorders, such as bursitis.

An occupational injury is "any injury such as a cut, fracture, sprain, amputation, and so on that results from a work-related accident or from an exposure involving a single incident in the work environment."

The determination of work-relatedness of an illness or injury is often difficult. Any exposure in the work environment is presumed to be work-related; however, exceptions to that rule exist as follows:
- An employee present in the work environment as a member of the general public
- Symptoms that occur at work as a result of a non–work-related event or exposure
- Voluntary participation in a wellness program, medical program, or fitness or recreational activity
- Ingestion of food for personal consumption, including that bought on the premises
- As a result of performing personal tasks at the workplace, outside working hours
- Activities of personal grooming, self-medication, or self-inflicted injuries
- Motor vehicle accident in an employer's parking lot or on an employer's access road while commuting to work
- Common colds or flu
- Mental illness

If it is not obvious whether an illness or injury is work related, the employee's job duties and work environment must be evaluated to determine whether an event or exposure caused or contributed to the condition or significantly aggravated a pre-existing condition.[12]

One type of incident is of particular concern to health care organizations: bloodborne pathogen exposures. For OSHA recordkeeping purposes, an occupational bloodborne pathogen exposure incident is classified as an injury, and is recorded if one of the following is true:
- The incident represents a work-related injury that involves loss of consciousness, transfer to another job, or restriction of work or motion.
- The incidents results in the recommendation of medical treatment beyond first aid, such as gamma globulin, hepatitis B immunoglobulin, hepatitis B vaccine, or zidovudine, regardless of dosage.

If a bloodborne pathogen exposure results in a seroconversion, the serological status of the employee is not reported to OSHA. This serves to protect the employee's confidentiality. If the seroconversion is known, it is recorded on the log as an injury (for example, as a needlestick). If known, the date of exposure is recorded. If multiple exposures are noted, the most recent date is recorded.

In some cases, called "privacy concern cases," it is not necessary to enter the employee's name on the 300 log. This provides the employee with confidentiality to encourage reporting. Events classified in this manner are
- Injury or illness to intimate body part or reproductive system
- Injury or illness resulting from sexual assault
- Mental illness
- HIV, hepatitis, or tuberculosis
- Needlesticks and sharp injuries

- Other illnesses, if independently and voluntarily requested

Another issue of importance to health care is tuberculosis (TB). A baseline tuberculin skin test should be performed on all new employees who are anticipated to have patient contact. A case of an employee diagnosed with TB should be recorded on the 300 log if that employee was exposed on the job to a known case of active tuberculosis and subsequently developed either an active TB infection or a positive tuberculin skin test. It would not be recorded if the employee was living in a household with a person diagnosed with active TB, the employee has been identified by the Public Health Department as a contact of an individual with active TB, or medical investigation shows that the employee's infection was caused by exposure away from work.

In addition to injuries and illnesses, organizations must report to OSHA any fatalities and/or catastrophes that take place in the work environment. Within eight hours of the event, an oral report must be made to OSHA of any work-related fatality, inpatient hospitalization of three or more employees, or fatal heart attack.

Conclusion

Developing a comprehensive and effective safety and health program requires multidisciplinary input from both leadership and staff. Risks should be anticipated and controls put in place to address the consequences of those risks. Open communication about risks and education and training can help build awareness among workers of the importance of safety. Both the Joint Commission and OSHA require organizations to take a hard look at themselves regarding worker safety and implement policies, procedures, and controls that make their facilities a safe place for employees to work. ∎

References

1. U.S. Department of Labor, Occupational Safety and Health Administration: *The Changing Workforce and Workplace.* http://www.osha.gov/oshinfo/strategic/pg2.html (accessed Jun. 20, 2003).

2. Maryland Occupational Safety and Health: *Developing a Workplace Safety and Health Program: A Program for Hazard Control.* http://www.dllr.state.md.us/labor/sandh/shprogcomp.html (accessed Jun. 21, 2003).

3. U.S. Department of Labor, Occupational Safety and Health Administration: *Draft Proposed Safety and Health Program Rule.* http://www.osha-slc.gov/SLTC/safetyhealth/nshp.html (accessed Mar. 18, 2005).

4. Tweedy J.T.: *Healthcare Hazard Control and Safety Management,* Boca Raton, Florida: GR/St. Lucie Press, 1997.

5. Bachman A.: *Six Steps to Safety: OSHA 2004 for Medical and Dental Practices.* Knoxville, TN: American Association of Physician Offices and Laboratories, 2004.

Chapter 1: OSHA Programs and Joint Commission Standards

6. Joint Commission Resources: Joint Commission, OSHA partnership aids health care compliance effort. *Environment of Care News* 4: 6-7, May/Jun. 2001.

7. Interview with Diana Ash, director of safety for Carolinas HealthCare System. Feb. 28, 2005.

8. U.S. Department of Labor: Occupational Safety and Health Administration: *Voluntary Protection Programs (VPP): Policies and Procedures Manual.* http://www.osha.gov/pls/oshaweb/owadisp.show_document?p_table=DIRECTIVES&p_id=2976#chapter6 (accessed Mar. 18, 2005).

9. Interview with Brenda Wehrle, vice president of quality/risk and Dorothy Lenz, employee/occupational health nurse for Blake Medical Center. Mar. 16, 2005.

10. U.S. Department of Labor: Occupational Safety and Health Administration: *Hazard Communication.* http://www.osha.gov/pls/oshaweb/owadisp.show_document?p_table=STANDARDS&p_id=10099 (accessed Mar. 18, 2005).

11. Joint Commission Resources: Cleaning up a mercury spill. *Environment of Care News* 6: 9-10, Jul. 2003.

12. U.S. Department of Labor: Occupational Safety and Health Administration: *Determination of Work-Relatedness.* http://www.osha.gov/pls/oshaweb/owadisp.show_document?p_table=STANDARDS&p_id=9636 (accessed Mar. 18, 2005).

Chapter 2:

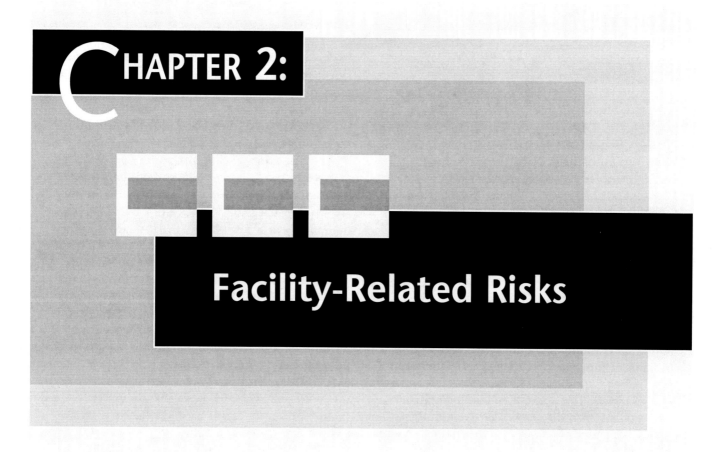

Facility-Related Risks

Some safety risks in the health care environment result from specific conditions or activities related to the facility. Several of these risks are present in nearly every environment. For example, what building is not at risk for fire or electrical hazards? Confined space found in elevator pits, sump pits, and boilers to be cleaned can all present potential hazards. Excessive noise can be a safety issue in some buildings depending on their location and layout. Asbestos can be found in almost any building that was built between the 1940s and the 1970s.

Still other risks found in general industry, such as those related to ventilation, have applications and concerns unique to health care. Ventilation issues are of significant concern to patients in health care facilities because of a heightened emphasis on infection control. But ventilation problems can have an effect on the staff members as well.

Confined Space

According to OSHA, confined spaces are areas that have limited or restricted means of entry and exit. They are large enough for employees to enter and perform their assigned work; however, they are not designed for continuous occupancy by employees. In health care organizations, commonly found confined spaces may include elevator pits, sump pits, boilers, utility tunnels, and water tanks. Individual buildings may have other unique spaces that would also fit into this category.

Confined spaces become potentially hazardous when another hazard is present in addition to the confined space. These hazards may include a hazardous atmosphere, a material that can potentially engulf the entrant, a recognized serious safety or health hazard, or an internal configuration such that an entrant might become entrapped or asphyxiated by inwardly converging walls or a floor that slopes downward[1].

Both the Joint Commission and OSHA require organizations to be cautious about confined spaces. Confined space entry is addressed implicitly in the Joint Commission standards under EC.1.10, EP1, which requires effective management of an environmental safety program for staff members and others in the facility. EC.1.20 requires that environmental tours are done annually for nonpatient care areas; potential confined spaces could be assessed as part of these tours in mechanical rooms and other similar locations.

STANDARDS: Joint Commission Standards that Implicitly Address Confined Spaces

- EC.1.10, Safety Management (EP1); EC.1.20, Environmental Tours
- HR.2.10, Initial Job Training; HR.2.20, Roles & Responsibilities; HR.2.30, Ongoing Education

OSHA provides detailed requirements addressing the issue of confined spaces. Their standard 29CFR 1910.146 requires organizations to control access to confined spaces via a permitting system with strict safeguards to provide for the safety of the entrant. Confined spaces that would fall under this requirement have another hazard in addition to the space itself.

Under OSHA's requirement, an employer must conduct an evaluation of the worksite to determine if any permit-required confined spaces exist in the work place. Employees must be notified if any of these spaces have been identified. This notification can be done with posted signage, such as

DANGER – PERMIT REQUIRED – CONFINED SPACE – AUTHORIZED ENTRANTS ONLY

and/or signage in other languages.

After any of these spaces have been identified, the next determination is whether employees will have to enter the spaces at any time to perform work. If so, a written program must be developed for permit-required confined spaces. Some of the things this written program must include are information on the hazards present in the space, measures to prevent unauthorized entry, specific job duties to be performed in the space, procedures for summoning rescue and emergency services, and written procedures for the permitting system for the space.

According to an annual analysis, confined spaces may be added to or removed from the list of permit-required spaces. It is evident that entry into one of these spaces must have a demonstrated need and a thorough evaluation. Clearly, it must be planned for well in advance of the actual entry.

Training

Both the Joint Commission and OSHA require employees to be properly trained prior to entering a permit-required confined space. Both organizations assess this training on the actual acquired knowledge of the employee. For example, the entrant of the confined space must know the hazards in the space and the signs and symptoms of exposure. He or she must know about appropriate personal protective equipment (PPE) and know how to use it properly. The attendant is a person who remains outside the space to monitor the entrant and assist in an emergency situation. Like the entrant, the attendant must be knowledgeable of the hazards and associated signs and symptoms of exposure. According to OSHA regulations, employees must receive a certificate of training from the employer that includes their name, signature or initials of the trainer(s), and the dates of training. Additional training is required with any changes in job duties, the program itself, the identification of new hazards, or any indication of employee need.

FIRE SAFETY

In health care organizations, fire is a unique risk related to the particular vulnerabilities of the patients involved. Fire is not only a facility-related risk; it can also flow into an evacuation scenario, which would be addressed under an organization's emergency management plan. While this chapter discusses fire safety in depth, more information on emergency plans can be found in Chapter Three.

The Joint Commission addresses fire safety in EC.5.10, with EP1 requiring a fire safety management plan and EP4 requiring a fire response plan to address the following issues:
- Facilitywide fire response
- Area-specific needs, including fire evacuation routes
- Specific roles and responsibilities of staff, licensed independent practitioners, and volunteers at a fire's point of origin
- Specific roles and responsibilities of staff, licensed independent practitioners, and volunteers away from a fire's point of origin
- Specific roles and responsibilities of staff, licensed independent practitioners, and volunteers in preparing for building evacuation

Chapter 2: Facility-Related Risks

STANDARDS: Joint Commission Standards that Address Fire Safety

- EC.1.10, Safety Management; EC.3.10, Hazardous Materials & Waste Management (7); EC.5.10, Fire Safety; EC.5.20, LSC Compliance; EC.5.30, Fire Drills; EC.5.40, Fire Safety Equipment; EC.5.50, Interim Life Safety Measures; EC.7.30, Utilities Maintenance
- HR.2.10, Initial Job Training; HR.2.20, Roles & Responsibilities; HR.2.30, Ongoing Education

Fire Prevention Plans

A written fire safety plan is required by Joint Commission for hospitals, ambulatory care, behavioral health care, long-term care organizations, and laboratories. OSHA requires that all workplaces with 10 or more employees write a fire safety plan. Those with fewer employees may communicate the plan orally.

Many of the requirements found in the Joint Commission Standards are also found within OSHA's requirements. Following is a discussion of OSHA's requirements and the corresponding Joint Commission requirements.

Within its requirements, OSHA describes the minimum elements that must be included in a fire prevention plan. One element is a list of all major fire hazards, proper handling and storage procedures for hazardous materials, potential ignition sources and their control, and the type of fire protection equipment necessary to control each major hazard [1910.39(c)(2)]².

The Joint Commission, in standard EC.5.20, requires health care organizations, as applicable by occupancy type, to be compliant with the 2000 edition of the National Fire Protection Association's *Life Safety Code®* (LSC). *

Furthermore, the Joint Commission requires organizations to complete a Statement of Conditions™ (SOC) document to assess code compliance. Any deficiencies identified by this process are to be recorded on a Plan for Improvement (PFI) with plans to correct them. Proper handling and storage of hazardous materials is found in the Joint Commission standards in EC.3.10 EP7, which requires the health care organization to provide "adequate and appropriate space and equipment for safely handling and storing hazardous materials and waste." Potential ignition sources would also be addressed in the *LSC* as well as EC.5.10 EP2, whereby the organization must proactively develop processes to protect individuals within facilities from fire, smoke, and other products of combustion. Fire protection equipment is specified in the LSC, with requirements for sprinkler and alarm systems. Fire extinguishers are placed in accordance with the OSHA standard on portable fire extinguishers, 29CFR 1910.157. Under EC.5.40, all the fire protection equipment is maintained, tested, and inspected.

Another element that OSHA requires in its fire prevention plans is procedures to control accumulations of flammable and combustible waste materials [1910.39(c)(2)]². These procedures are addressed by the Joint Commission under the requirement to be compliant with the LSC in applicable organizations. Even business occupancies, which are not required by the Joint Commission to be LSC compliant, are expected to be maintained in a fire-safe condition. Furthermore, during construction activities, one of the interim life safety measures (ILSM) that may be implemented to compensate for an LSC deficiency under EC.5.50 is "developing and enforcing storage, housekeeping, and debris removal practices that reduce the building's flammable and combustible fire load to the lowest feasible level."

OSHA also requires a fire safety plan to contain procedures for regular maintenance of safeguards installed on heat-producing equipment to prevent the accidental ignition of combustible materials [1910.39(c)(3)]².

The Joint Commission addresses this issue within the preventive maintenance requirements of EC.7.30. Many organizations issue "hot work permits" for certain specified jobs, such as welding. Under a permitting system, the organization is knowledgeable as to the activities that are taking place to ensure that they are conducted safely. In addition, certain heat-producing equipment, such as space heaters, are often prohibited within health care organizations to reduce the risk of fire.

As with all types of hazards, the Joint Commission and OSHA want employees to be aware of any fire hazards to which they are exposed. The Joint Commission requires orientation and ongoing education about safety in HR.2.10, HR.2.20, and HR.2.30 in the Human Resources chapter of the accreditation manuals; this includes education about fire hazards and emergency management. OSHA requires employers to provide information to their employees about the fire hazards to which they are exposed in the workplace. The fire prevention plan should be reviewed with employees upon initial assignment to a job.

---

* *Life Safety Code®* is a registered trademark of the National Fire Protection Association, Quincy, MA.

Business Occupancies

Health care organizations classified by the Joint Commission as business occupancies are not required to be compliant with the LSC. They are, however, required to be maintained in a fire-safe condition. A business occupancy is a facility where no one stays overnight and three or fewer people are rendered incapable of self-preservation at any one time by the care or treatment provided there. Even though these organizations do not need to comply with the LSC, they still must have clear and safe exit routes. According to OSHA, an "exit route" is defined as "a continuous and unobstructed path of exit travel from any point within a workplace to a place of safety (including refuge areas). An exit route consists of three parts: the exit access, the exit, and the exit discharge. (An exit route includes all vertical and horizontal areas along this route.)"[3] The design, construction, maintenance, safeguards, and operational features for exit routes are all covered under OSHA's standards (29CFR 1910.36 and 29CFR 1910.37). Organizations that are deemed business occupancies should review these standards to ensure compliance.

Control of Hazardous Energy and Electrical Safety

Hazardous energy sources can be found in many, if not most, pieces of mechanical or electrical equipment used in health care organizations. Any source of mechanical, hydraulic, pneumatic, chemical, thermal, or other energy falls into this classification.

The Joint Commission addresses electrical safety in several areas. Environment of Care (EC) standards discuss the development and maintenance of an effective environmental safety program including the inspection, testing, and maintenance of fire protection equipment, medical equipment, and components of utility systems. This implies that electrical safety will be considered and attended to appropriately.

STANDARDS *Joint Commission Standards that Implicitly Address Hazardous Energy and Electrical Safety*

▶ EC.1.10, Safety Management; EC.5.40, Fire Safety Equipment; EC.6.20, Medical Equipment Maintenance
▶ HR.2.10, Initial Job Training; HR.2.20, Roles & Responsibilities; HR.2.30, Ongoing Education

---

As with many areas of worker safety, OSHA is prescriptive in their requirements.

While the Joint Commission does not require compliance with OSHA standards, they are discussed here for consideration.

There is one OSHA regulation addressing Lockout/Tagout: 29CFR 1910.147, *Control of Hazardous Energy*. Along with the standard is Appendix A, which provides a sample lockout procedure. Other OSHA regulations address a broad spectrum of electrical safety issues, grouped by topic:

- Protective equipment (29CFR 1910.137)
- Electric power (29CFR 1910.269)
- Design safety standards for electrical systems (29CFR 1910.302–1910.308)
- Safety-related work practices (29CFR 1910.331–1910.335)

Many of these electrical safety standards are applicable to health care facilities, and they include highly technical information specific to the application. Individuals working with these applications are advised to refer directly to these regulations. The general design safety standard, 1910.303, will be addressed below.

OSHA's general requirements for electrical design safety standards address a variety of basic issues. The ultimate goal of these standards is to ensure that electrical equipment is free from recognized hazards that are likely to cause death or serious physical harm to employees.[4] OSHA includes several considerations to determine the safety of the equipment:

Suitability for installation and use in conjunction with OSHA requirements, which may be accomplished by listing or labeling the equipment's purpose
- Mechanical strength and durability
- Electrical insulation
- Heating effects when in use
- Arcing effects
- Classification by type, size, voltage, current capacity, specific use[4]

OSHA standards require electrical equipment to be marked with the manufacturer's name and trademark or other marking. Voltage, current, wattage, or other ratings should also be marked on the equipment. Other safety considerations addressed in OSHA's standards include working space around electrical equipment, ensuring appropriate clearances, and access to working space and headroom. Appropriate lighting must be provided for all working spaces for service equipment, switchboards, panelboards, and motor control centers.

Lockout/Tagout

Workers maintaining or servicing equipment that is still energized are at risk of exposure to energy sources if the equipment starts up or releases energy unexpectedly during their task. The regulations and standards related to the control of this hazardous energy to prevent worker exposure are commonly known as Lockout/Tagout.

OSHA defines "lockout" as "the placement of a lockout device on an energy-isolating device, in accordance with an established procedure, ensuring that the energy-isolating device and the equipment being controlled cannot be operated until the lockout device is removed." In short, a physical device that prevents harmful energizing is applied to the equipment.

"Tagout" is "the placement of a tagout device on an energy-isolating device, in accordance with an established procedure, to indicate that the energy-isolating device and the equipment being controlled may not be operated until the tagout device is removed." A "tagout device" is "any prominent warning device, such as a tag and a means of attachment that can be securely fastened to an energy-isolating device to indicate that the machine or equipment to which it is attached may not be operated until the tagout device is removed."[5] Lockout is always preferable to tagout when feasible. Although a lockout device physically prevents energizing equipment, a tagout device only warns against it.

OSHA's lockout/tagout standard applies to any energy source and most activities where the workers could be exposed to an unanticipated startup of the equipment or a release of hazardous energy. This includes constructing, installing, adjusting, inspecting, cleaning activities, and others.

Service and maintenance activities that are performed during normal operation of the equipment are covered under the requirements if the employee must remove safety devices, such as guarding, or the worker is required to place a body part into a point of operation or a danger zone of the machine. Servicing and maintenance are not covered if the safeguards in place are effective in preventing exposure to the energy hazards.

Other noncovered activities include minor tool changes and adjustments, assuming the effective protection of workers. Work on electrical equipment that is connected with a cord or plug is excluded if the equipment is unplugged and the worker has exclusive control of the plug. Hot tap operations that involve transmission and distribution systems for gas, steam, water, or petroleum products on pressurized pipelines are not covered if continuity of the service is critical and it is impractical to shut down the system. In this case, procedures must be followed and employees must use appropriate protection.

Energy Control Program

Under the OSHA standards, an employer is required to develop an energy control program for any covered activities to ensure that the equipment being serviced is isolated from the energy source and is therefore inoperative. Specifically, logout/tagout procedures must be addressed in this program. The program must consist of procedures, periodic inspections, and employee training.

Procedures

The procedures for energy control must provide the information that the employee servicing the equipment needs, including the purpose, rule, and techniques to accomplish lockout/tagout. Employers may develop their own procedures to meet their particular needs; however, OSHA has some content specifications as follows:

- Scope, purpose, authorization, rules, techniques
- Means to enforce compliance
- Statement of intended use
- Steps to shut down, isolate, block, and secure equipment
- Steps for placement, removal, and transfer of lockout or tagout devices and a description of who has responsibility for them
- Requirements to test equipment to verify the effectiveness of the lockout and tagout devices and other control measures[5]

Inspection

OSHA requires inspection of an organization's lockout/tagout procedures at least annually. This inspection must be completed by an authorized employee who is not involved in the procedure being inspected. Any deficiencies must be identified and corrected. Each authorized employee involved in lockout procedures must participate in a review of his or her responsibilities. In procedures using tagout, the inspector must review the authorized and the effected employees' responsibilities. The employer is required to certify that the inspection took place, including the identification of the machine, the date of the inspection, the participating employees, and the individual who performed the inspection.

Training

Training requirements depend on the category of the employee, and training must be performed before the employee participates in a lockout/tagout procedure. Training for employees who are servicing equipment should include recognition of applicable energy sources, type and magnitude of energy available in the workplace and methods and means for energy isolation and control.

Training for employees using the equipment should include the purpose and use of the lockout/tagout procedure. Other employees who may not work in the affected area must still be trained about the procedure and the prohibition of attempts to restart equipment that is locked out or tagged out.

As previously stated, tags are to be used only if locks are not feasible. Therefore, if a tagout system is used, employees must be trained on the limitation of tags. Such limitations may include the following:

- Tags are warning devices only and do not physically prevent the activation of the equipment.
- Tags must not be removed without authorization and must never be bypassed or ignored.
- Tags must be legible and understandable.
- Tags and the means of their attachment must be made of materials that will stand up to workplace environmental conditions.
- The meaning of tags must be understood so that they do not give a false sense of security.
- Tags must be securely attached so they cannot accidentally become detached.[5]

VENTILATION

Heating, ventilating, and air conditioning (HVAC) systems provide circulating air throughout health care facilities. They provide temperature and humidity control and filtration of various contaminants. The rationale for Joint Commission EC.7.10 calls for a safe, controlled, and comfortable environment, and these utility systems components are to a large extent responsible for that type of environment. When HVAC systems aren't functioning optimally, they can be a source of workplace safety hazards, as well as hazards for patients and all others in the facility.

Standards and Regulations

The Joint Commission has a variety of standards related to ventilation and indoor air quality. EC.7.10 is one of the core standards for the topic. It requires organizations to ensure that the utilities management program "reduces the potential for organization-acquired illness to be transmitted through the utility systems." Organization-acquired illness, or health care–associated infections (per guidelines) (HAIs), is usually thought of as a problem impacting patients within health care facilities. But poor air quality and the transmission of airborne contaminants can affect employees as well. EP16 of that standard specifically addresses the issue of air quality in areas aimed at protecting the most vulnerable patients. It requires organization to design, install, and maintain ventilation equipment to provide appropriate pressure relationships, air-exchange rates, and filtration efficiencies for ventilation systems for these areas. While this standard is focused on preserving the safety of the most vulnerable patients, the standard also protects staff who may be vulnerable to infection or susceptible to allergies.

Further in the standards, the Joint Commission addresses temperature and humidity. Standard EC.8.10, EP7 states, "Ventilation provides for acceptable levels of temperature and humidity and eliminates odors." This directly relates to indoor air quality and potentially to sick building syndrome and/or building-related illness.

Finally, EC.8.30 requires the performance of a pre-construction risk assessment to be done from the planning stages of any project involving construction, demolition, or renovation within the health care facility. This assessment must address the impact on air quality, infection control, and utility requirements, as well as other issues. Controls must be identified and implemented to reduce and minimize the impact of the construction activities. Most often this assessment is based on the location of particularly vulnerable patients, but staff must be considered too.

STANDARDS *Joint Commission Standards that Address Ventilation*

➤ EC.1.20, Environmental Tours; EC.7.10, Utilities Management (EP16); EC.7.30, Utilities Maintenance; EC.8.10, Appropriate Environment (EP7); EC.8.30, Built Environment; EC.9.10, Monitoring Environmental Conditions; EC.9.20, Analyzing Environmental Issues

---

OSHA addresses ventilation issues in several standards. Some of these are more applicable to health care than others. For example, indoor air quality issues are of sig-

Chapter 2: Facility-Related Risks

nificant importance to health care organizations. Those OSHA standards that address permissible exposure limits for various chemicals (see Chapter 1, Hazard Communication) do relate to ventilation, because the level of contaminant present can be reduced by increased ventilation of the area. Despite discussion of the importance of proper ventilation with regard to worker safety, there are no specific OSHA regulations relating to ventilation and indoor air quality.

Indoor Air Quality

The American Society of Heating, Refrigerating, and Air-Conditioning Engineers (ASHRAE), states that high-quality indoor air is "air in which there are no known contaminants at harmful concentrations as determined by cognizant authorities and with which a substantial majority (80% or more) of the people exposed do not express dissatisfaction."

Other, slightly different definitions are available. Klingelsmith defines high-quality indoor air as "an indoor environmental condition that contains the lowest possible level of a broad scope of air pollutants to satisfy the health, comfort, and well being of the vast majority of occupants in any type of building at any given time."[6] Baril says that high-quality indoor air is "the physical, biological, and chemical characteristics of indoor air that affect the comfort or health of the occupant."[7]

The common element of these three definitions is the subjective opinions of the buildings' occupants, which cannot be objectively defined. Characteristics of good indoor air quality (IAQ), however, can be identified:
- Adequate ventilation
- Comfortable temperature and humidity
- Air movement
- Preventive maintenance of systems
- Control of construction contaminants

IAQ concerns date back to the 1970s. The energy crisis of that era resulted in the construction of tighter buildings with the intent to minimize energy consumption and therefore costs. Buildings were better insulated and less outdoor air was used. Filters rated at only 10% – 20% efficiency were installed to create low pressure drops, but they also allowed the passage of particles.

Other cost concerns at the time reduced or eliminated the commissioning of some HVAC systems, and maintenance may have been deferred. According to Burroughs, "Systems, situations, loads, usages, efficiencies, and costs all change over time. As buildings age, they wear, deteriorate, leak, break, and fail."[8] Therefore, sound maintenance and operations of the HVAC system are critical.

Air Handling and Ventilation Systems

Airborne contaminants include biological agents—bacteria, viruses, and molds—as well as gases, fumes, and dust. The primary means of controlling such contaminants in health care organizations is the design, installation, and maintenance of an HVAC system.

The Joint Commission recommends that organizations involve design professionals who are appropriately credentialed and adhere to specifications contained in state and local codes and in guidelines available from ASHRAE and in the *Guidelines for Design and Construction of Hospitals and Health Care Facilities,* pubished by the American Institute of Architects (AIA).

From the perspective of all these organizations and the Joint Commission, HVAC systems pose three areas of infection control concern:
- Pressure relationships (whether air flows from corridor to room or vice versa)
- Air exchange rates (dilution of contaminants)
- Filtration efficiencies (removal of particulates)

These variables all work together efficiently in an effective environmental infection control program.

The particulars of an organization's ventilation policies will depend on what types of procedures the organization performs, what types of patients it serves, and of course what kinds of organisms it identifies. Different areas might require different levels of temperature, humidity, velocity, and filtration.

Pressure Relationships

Pressure differential is a measure of air velocity. Pressure control via an offset between supply air and exhaust air volumes is essential in keeping airborne contaminants from migrating into critical areas.

The *AIA Guidelines* specify the use of negative air pressure in emergency department (ED) triage and waiting areas and in radiology departments, and positive pressure in outpatient surgery suites when not in use. The guidelines also prescribe reversible pressure in isolation rooms and recommend that organizations measure pressure differentials in these rooms using visual monitoring of airflow into airborne infectious isolation (AII) rooms, and smoke tubes, flutter strips, or other simple devices to measure airflow out of protective environment rooms. The *AIA Guidelines* permit the use of high-efficiency particulate air (HEPA) filters to clean the air before recirculation as a way to offset the extra energy costs associated with exhausting AII air directly to the outside.

EC staff will want to monitor air pressurization in

the previously mentioned rooms, which must be well sealed and supplied with emergency power to ensure continuous operation of ventilation systems. Staff should also routinely maintain and calibrate sensors and monitoring devices.

Air Exchange Rates

In most locations, health codes allow a reduction in minimum total airflow rates and minimum outdoor airflow rates during unoccupied periods, thus allowing hospitals—which typically occupy only 15% – 20% of their space constantly—to realize significant energy savings by using variable air volume (VAV) tracking systems. The AIA and ASHRAE allow ventilation rates to be reduced to 25% of the occupied period rates, as long as continuous directional control and space pressurization is maintained at all times and the full (occupied) ventilation air change rates can be reestablished at any time.

Filtration

Filtration is the primary defense against fungi in ventilation systems. HEPA filters might not be necessary; prefilters are effective against most fungi, even when in spore form, provided the filters are tightly installed and well maintained. It is important to note that fungi can grow in the filters as well.

Many health care facilities these days must struggle with staff cutbacks, which often affect environmental services. Where this situation exists, it is up to the facility manager and the infection control professionals to jointly make the case for spending additional money on HEPA filters or increased air exchanges in areas at greatest risk.

Maintenance

Fans, coils, belts, and filters all require regular maintenance to function properly. Organizations should establish preventive maintenance, cleaning, and inspection schedules for the HVAC system and stick to them. It is also important to keep accurate, up-to-date records of not only routine maintenance but also requested maintenance and quality management activities, including the use of instrumentation to determine appropriate air change, filtration, and pressure parameters for areas requiring special ventilation.

Following are some common maintenance tasks for air distribution systems in health care organizations:
- Change filters when a manometer reading indicates they are full
- Adjust louvers and dampers for air balance
- Keep automatic controls in good working order
- Thoroughly clean ducts if they become contaminated
- Change pulleys and belts as needed
- Clean screens and keep them tight
- Periodically calibrate and test negative pressure alarms
- Do not allow birds and other creatures to contaminate inlets and other building systems

Reviewing and approving engineering and maintenance polices and procedures related to inspections and preventive maintenance of utility systems is one area where organizations should get input from both facilities management and infection control.[9]

All the above-described characteristics of a health care ventilation system come into focus when an organization faces an infectious disease outbreak. Several Canadian hospitals saw this first-hand with the 2003 outbreak of Severe Acute Respiratory Syndrome (SARS). The case study on this page illustrates the experience. In addition, health care organizations in the United States are benefiting from Canada's experience. This can be seen in the case study on page 34.

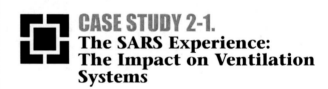

CASE STUDY 2-1.
The SARS Experience: The Impact on Ventilation Systems

One of Canada's largest health care facilities, Sunnybrook & Women's (S&W), is a 1,400-bed tertiary/quaternary center that is an amalgam of three separate hospitals located around Toronto. During SARS l, S&W screened thousands of staff and visitors daily for SARS and managed more than 70 inpatients, the largest volume of in-hospital SARS patients outside mainland China.

Additional pressures were placed on S&W as other facilities closed due to SARS outbreaks. As the largest trauma center in the country, S&W treated almost all the trauma patients in the greater Toronto area and saw a significant increase in the number of emergency department visits.

The hospital's Director of Facilities Services, Harry Taylor, recalled that "When SARS first hit, we knew very little about the disease. But it quickly became evident that our number

Chapter 2: Facility-Related Risks

one priority had to be creating negative pressure rooms." The hospital chose to dedicate a general medicine floor as a SARS unit and almost overnight turned the 22 rooms in that unit into negative pressure rooms.

In newer isolation rooms, an automatic alarm indicates when the room loses negative pressure. But S&W couldn't afford the time to buy and install those monitoring units. So facilities engineers set up a testing program to make sure the rooms were, in fact, staying negative. "Each day our technicians performed smoke testing to show which way the air was flowing," said Taylor. "And each day they would see smoke disappear underneath the door of the patient rooms, indicating that all was well with the negative pressure."

In their concern about ensuring negative air pressure, S&W filtered the exhaust through HEPA filters that would screen out any harmful elements. The hospital purchased 22 portable units from a supplier in Quebec. "When we told them how critical the situation was," said Taylor, "they shipped the filters overnight, and we had them installed in less than 24 hours."

The hospital was also the first health care facility in Toronto to create a SARS assessment unit where symptomatic community residents could come to the emergency department to be evaluated for possible SARS. To accomplish this, S&W set up nearly 5,000 square feet of space at its Women's College Ambulatory Care Centre about five miles from the main campus and staffed it with doctors, nurses, and security officers. This was an important strategy to keep potential SARS patients away from the main facility.

Taylor points out that, in coping with an emergency such as SARS, facilities managers play a vital role and can draw on a wealth of resources. In addition to their own staff, they have access to engineering groups, suppliers, and peer groups at other hospitals. Taylor's advice to other facilities management people who might someday face a similar challenge: "Be a strategic resource for your organization and work closely with your senior leadership team. Educate people on the technical aspects of the building environment. Help in the development of tactical strategies, and then execute your plans quickly." U.S. hospitals following Joint Commission emergency management standards (EC.4.10) will be completing a hazard vulnerability analysis to identify in advance potential emergencies that could affect the need for their services or their ability to provide those services. This would be an opportunity to set up pre-established supplier relationships for the identified vulnerabilities.

SARS also allowed S&W to test its ability to respond to a large-scale emergency. "S&W did an amazing job in pulling together," said Taylor. "It was stressful for everyone in the hospital, but the 400 people on our facilities management team—plant operations, environmental services, security, and our parking and transportation group—never hesitated for an instant to do what was needed. In fact, some of our people volunteered to take on tasks that would require them to be quarantined at work and at home."

Following is a list of recommendations for hospital facilities managers culled from suggestions made by Lucy Brun, a Toronto-area health care and infectious disease expert, and Susan Kwolek, vice president of quality and corporate performance at Toronto's North York General Hospital, a 434-bed facility that dealt with the second phase of the SARS outbreak:

- Provide sufficient surge capacity to address emergencies
- Reduce the number of entry/exit points to the facility; control access via cameras and swipe cards
- Separate the hospital's "mission-critical" departments and access to these areas
- Implement mechanical and ventilation systems to support isolation and separation of air intakes and exhaust
- Provide adequate individual space per patient; for example, more than four feet from one patient/visitor face to the next patient/visitor face
- Keep an adequate supply of PPE (face masks, gloves, gowns, and so on) on hand at all times and make sure that those supplies are readily available
- Clean patient units on every shift
- Clean all facilities and equipment that are in common use; for example, nursing stations, computer keyboards, telephones, and so on
- Use basic infection control methods as outlined in Joint Commission standards for the Surveillance, Prevention, and Control of Infection, in the applicable accreditation manual[10]

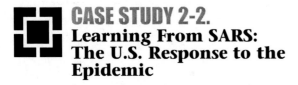

CASE STUDY 2-2.
Learning From SARS: The U.S. Response to the Epidemic

Skip Gregory, bureau chief of the Office of Plans and Construction at Florida's Agency for Health Care Administration, reports that the Agency is currently investigating how to expand the surge capacity of Florida hospitals to cope with infectious disease outbreaks. Hospitals are being alerted to deal with the following scenarios:

- How to manipulate the hospital's HVAC system to turn patient rooms into negative pressure air rooms and exhaust the infectious air to the outside without returning it to the building
- How to find products that can be affixed to walls or ceilings to convert normal patient rooms into negative pressure air rooms
- How to set up a temporary structure within a designated area of the community that would enable a certain segment of the population to be isolated

And a working group at Tampa General Hospital has submitted the following proposed guidelines for arresting or preventing a disease outbreak to the Florida Hospital Association for review by and input from other hospitals throughout the state. The hope is eventually to enact these recommendations to regulate patient placement and movement in the event of a disease outbreak. The facility will do the following:

- Accommodate 10 beds
- Provide negative air pressure in relation to surrounding areas; minimum of one one-hundredth (.01) of an inch
- Provide a magnahelic gauge to ensure that pressure differentials are maintained
- Monitor continuously for negative air pressure
- Provide at least 12 air changes per hour of circulation (supply and exhaust)
- Ensure that air is exhausted to the outdoors on the roof of the facility through monitored HEPA filters; no air from this facility will be circulated to other areas
- Provide supply air that is conditioned for summer or winter
- Provide automatic door closers to ensure that doors are closed
- Provide anterooms with air supply to maintain positive air pressure
- Provide medical gas (oxygen, vacuum, and medical air) at each bed
- Provide an emergency power supply to critical medical equipment and air circulation equipment
- Provide hand-cleaning facilities and toilet facilities[10]

Sick Building Syndrome

Sick Building Syndrome (SBS) is the terminology used to describe a condition believed to be caused by a building that is considered to be contaminated. SBS is a physical reaction to various types of low-level contaminants, which may or may not pose an actual health risk. Therefore, investigation and management of SBS issues must distinguish perception from true risk.

SBS occurs when a health care facility's systems aren't functioning properly and elements in the indoor air environment affect the health of workers and patients. The generic cause of SBS is an elevation of one or more of the following types of contaminants to a potentially harmful level:

- Airborne dust and inorganic particulate matter
- Airborne volatile organic chemicals and vapors
- Allergens, pollens, environmental mold, and bacteria[9]

The symptoms of SBS are vague, involving nonspecific upper-respiratory discomfort, such as chest tightness, sore throat, coughing, runny nose, burning or itching eyes, headache, lethargy, and fatigue. These symptoms are common to many human maladies, and are often assumed to be the flu or the like. If they actually are SBS symptoms, they will persist for an extended period of time.

The very nature of SBS is that the symptoms will abate or disappear when the affected individual leaves the building. Discomfort, irritation, and attendant deterioration in productivity are brought about by a prolonged exposure to air constituents that occur normally in low or modest concentrations.

SBS Causes

The following elements are believed to contribute to the poor IAQ that causes SBS. These elements can be exacerbated by humidity or extremes in temperature.

- Chemical contaminants from outdoor sources: Outdoor air that enters a building can become a source of indoor pollution. Vapors from motor vehicle exhaust, plumbing vents, and building exhausts can enter the building through improperly located air intake vents, windows, and other openings. One hospital solved an IAQ problem by raising to roof level an air intake formerly located at ground level near the ambulance entrance.
- Chemical contaminants from indoor sources: Most indoor pollution comes from sources inside the building. Adhesives, upholstery, carpeting, copy machines, manufactured wood products, cleaning agents, and pesticides can emit volatile organic compounds (VOCs), including formaldehyde. At high concentrations, some VOCs can cause chronic acute health effects, and some are known carcinogens. Tobacco smoke, cleaning and maintenance products, synthetic fragrances in personal care products and combustion products from stoves can send chemical contaminants into the air.
- Biological contaminants: These contaminants—including pollen, bacteria, viruses, and molds—can breed in stagnant water that has accumulated in humidifiers, drain pans, and ducts or on ceiling tiles, insulation, or carpeting. Biological contaminants can cause fever, chills, cough, chest tightness, muscle aches, and allergic reactions.
- Inadequate ventilation: Contemporary building energy efficiency has been improved by making buildings more airtight, with less outdoor air ventilation. In many cases, these reduced outdoor ventilation rates make workers uncomfortable and prone to illness.[9]

Prevention of SBS

In addition to increasing ventilation rates and air distribution, organizations can take one or more of the following steps:

- Take special care with special spaces: Specially designed areas include spaces such as operating rooms, special procedure rooms, delivery rooms, rooms for patients diagnosed or suspected of having airborne communicable diseases (for example, pulmonary or laryngeal tuberculoses; see Chapter Four), rooms for patients requiring protective isolation (for example, those receiving bone marrow transplants), laboratories, pharmacies, and sterile supply rooms.
- Monitor how space is used: If part of a facility built for a specific purpose is later used for a different purpose, the ventilation system might not be appropriate. This point is especially important in older buildings that have been updated or renovated many times. When you change the way a space is used, for example, using a different type of equipment in a room or on a floor, the HVAC system should be changed to accommodate the new use.
- Remove or modify pollutants: Removing or modifying pollutant sources is the most effective way to eliminate a known source of an air quality problem. Ways to do so include performing routine maintenance of HVAC systems; replacing water-stained ceiling tiles and carpets; venting source emissions to the outdoors; storing paints, solvents, pesticides, and adhesives in closed containers in well-ventilated areas; and allowing time for building materials in new or remodeled areas to off-gas pollutants before occupying those areas.
- Clean air: This tactic is a useful supplement to source control and ventilation, but it has limitations. Particle control devices such as furnace filters are inexpensive but do not capture small particles effectively. High-performance air filters capture small particles but are relatively expensive to install and operate. Some gaseous pollutants might be removed by absorbent beds, but these devices can be expensive and the absorbent material must be replaced often.
- Ensure that housekeeping is done properly: If operations, housekeeping, and maintenance tasks aren't performed correctly, mold can grow on wet building materials. The housekeeping staff should be instructed to dry spills immediately before mold can accumulate. A good rule of thumb is that if it can't be completely dried within three days, it should be removed.
- Check the mechanical system: A poorly designed mechanical system—or one that has been modified so drastically that it doesn't meet a building's current requirements—can lead to SBS. Those systems are designed to maintain the proper balance, the proper filtration, and air pressures; if you're not maintaining the system, it might not be performing up to the original standards for which it was designed.
- Educate and communicate: Education and communication are essential for preventive and remedial indoor air quality management programs. Key individuals should know the basics of air quality issues and the facility's plans for handling them. Education on air quality is just as important for administrators and clinical staff as it is for facilities and safety departments. When all employees communicate effectively and

understand the causes and consequences of air quality problems, they can work together to prevent problems from occurring.[9]

Building related illnesses (BRI) are similar to SBS, and organizations should be aware of and try to prevent these as well. BRIs are said to occur when clinical proof that an illness is related to a building is found. Types of illnesses that may be considered BRI include:
- Allergies
- Fungal infections
- Bacterial infections
- Viral infections
- Legionnaire's Disease (see Chapter Five)

Approximately 95% of infections acquired in health care organizations are from direct contact; however, the remaining 5% are airborne, and therefore under the influence of the management of the facility and its HVAC system.

Controlling Airborne Contaminants

With respect to indoor air quality controls, one must keep in mind that there are no permissible exposure limits for pathogenic indoor contaminants. Many of the contaminants inside a health care building occur naturally outside. In addition, members of the building population are potential carriers of some pathogens.

Airborne contaminants that must be controlled are biological agents, which include bacteria, molds, and fungi, as well as gases, fumes, and dust. Other concerns are volatile organic compounds, allergens, and irritants. Volatile organic compounds are frequently irritants associated with the off-gassing of new carpeting or upholstered furniture. These compounds may also be associated with the use of glutaraldehyde, formaldehyde, xylene, paint, caulk, or adhesives.

Allergens may stem from insects, rodents, dander, laboratory animals, and so forth. Their impact is dependent on individual sensitivities, and there are no permissible exposure limits. The American College of Government Industrial Hygienists (ACGIH) recommends levels that are less than one-third of the outdoor levels. Fungi, such as *Aspergillus sp.*, grow on cellulose-based materials such as gypsum board and ceiling tiles, and it is therefore imperative that any of these materials that have become wet are either thoroughly dried within 72 hours or removed and replaced. Fungal spores become airborne very easily after being disturbed, and care must be taken to carefully wet any affected material before its removal so that spores do not become airborne. Sources of fungi include outdoor air, construction dust, excavation, wet areas in the HVAC system, living plants, and bird and bat droppings. For example, health care facilities must be very conscientious in controlling the local pigeon population to avoid the spread of *Histoplasma sp.* contained in their droppings.

In health care facilities, airborne bacteria can be spread through the HVAC system. An example of this type of contamination would be *Mycobacterium tuberculosis,* the bacterium responsible for causing TB. TB is spread via "droplet nuclei," which are droplets containing the bacteria. The droplets become airborne when an infected patient coughs, sneezes, or even speaks or sings. (See Chapter Four for more detailed information on tuberculosis.)

Controls

Engineering controls associated with improved indoor air quality include general dilution ventilation. The more clean air that is circulated into a space, the less the impact of any contaminants. Space pressurization is used to ensure that air movement is directed from a clean space into a less-clean space. HEPA filtration can be used to remove small airborne particles.

The primary means of controlling airborne contaminants are the design, installation, and maintenance of the heating, ventilation, and air conditioning system. Design professionals who are appropriately credentialed should be involved with the process, and guidelines from professional organizations should be used, such as those from
- ASHRAE (American Society of Heating, Refrigerating, and Air Conditioning Engineers)
- State and/or local codes
- American Institute of Architects (AIA) *Guidelines for Design and Construction of Hospital and Health Care Facilities*

Pressure gradients and air exchange rates should be designed and set according to the services performed and individuals served in various areas of the building. A good source of information for these settings is the AIA *Guidelines*. (Note, however, that the AIA *Guidelines* document specifically applies to new construction only, and the recommendations contained therein may not be achievable in existing facilities.) After these settings are appropriately verified, air balancing does not have to be regularly performed unless the system is modified or breached.

Chapter 2: Facility-Related Risks

Preventive maintenance, cleaning, and inspection schedules for the HVAC system should be prudently established and strictly followed for parts such as fans, coils, belts, and filters. Proper fit of filters is essential to their effective functioning. A related issue is the inspecting, testing, and maintaining of the negative pressure rooms for suspected or confirmed tuberculosis.[11]

In the *OSHA Technical Manual* for health hazards in hospitals[12], some important points are made about local ventilation engineering controls as follows:

- "Hoods should be used for specific procedures, such as mixing antineoplastic drugs. A scavenging system that contains a proper gas disposal system must be in place and operable."
- "Portable suction devices may be used for direct removal of contaminants. Portable ventilation should be used for smoke plume removal during laser surgery."
- "Ethylene oxide should be ventilated through a nonrecycled or dedicated ventilation system."
- "In the morgue, local vacuum systems should be in place for power saws."
- "Mixing of methyl methacrylate should be done in a closed system."

These points contribute to the reduction of various airborne contaminants and/or odors.

IAQ Program

When setting up an IAQ program, organizations may want to consider the following actions:

- Organize the IAQ program team, and designate one person to be in charge of the program. Team members may include (where applicable) representatives of engineering, architecture, construction management, employee safety, infection control, human resources, and risk management.
- Gather all mechanical system and facility-related documents such as building plans, submittal data, equipment lists, air balancing reports, and material safety data sheets. Include equipment maintenance logs as they relate to IAQ.
- Write a short description of the facility, including the original construction date and the dates of all additions and expansions. Include a description of the current HVAC system and its major components.
- Write an action plan for dealing with IAQ complaints.

Indoor Air Quality Investigation

As stated previously, reports of IAQ issues may be perceived rather than real. However, all complaints should be investigated to avoid developing hostility and to maintain confidence in management's support for a safe environment.

Odor complaints may be especially nebulous. An unpleasant smell that may or may not pose a health threat might exist. Many odor complaints may be managed by dilution ventilation. An assessment of the location of air intakes with respect to prevailing winds should be included in the investigation of these complaints. Leaks in the plumbing vent system may result in sulfur dioxide or hydrogen sulfide odors. Communication with staff members is particularly important in these investigations.[13]

Education and Training

IAQ is an often-misunderstood topic, and the only way to gain a comfortable level of understanding when dealing with IAQ-related issues is through education and training. Health care facilities should provide basic education to all employees, not just those with responsibility for compliance and correction.

Employee training could include the signs and symptoms of BRI and the procedure to report complaints. Employees should understand that there is a facility plan for dealing with these issues, and that all reports and concerns will be investigated. Those who are responsible for operating and maintaining the utility systems should be provided with appropriate training in the procedures and associated use of PPE.[13]

The case study on this page discusses how one organization developed a structure appropriate to IAQ managements, specifically addressing the issues of moisture and bioaerosols management.

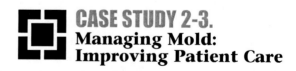

CASE STUDY 2-3.
Managing Mold: Improving Patient Care

Kaiser Permanente Develops a Standardized Approach

Molds occur naturally in the environment and are an essential part of the world's ecosystems. Without mold, the world would be overwhelmed with large amounts of dead plant matter. Mold is critical to the breakdown of leaves, wood, and other plant debris.

But mold can also grow indoors when moisture accumulates from sources such as pipe leaks, roof leaks, or condensation. While outdoor mold is good, indoor mold growth can be a problem. When molds grow inside a building, sensitive individuals such as those with compromised immune systems, allergies to mold, and other medical conditions can have adverse reactions. Such sensitive individuals are usually present in health care organizations.

Why Address Mold?

In 2004, Kaiser Permanente, a large health maintenance organization that owns and operates its own medical centers, saw a need to standardize its approach to mold management. Both the Association for Professionals in Infection Control and Epidemiology (APIC) and the AIA had issued guidance documents addressing the need for organizations to control dust, thus reducing infection risks on a wholesale level. A large portion of dust contains mold spores. Kaiser felt that an integral part of dust control was mold management. "There has been a lot of media hype around mold, but very little regulatory attention to the issue. While mold is not acceptable inside an organization, it is a manageable risk, the treatment of which should be straightforward," stated Tim Havel, director of the Western Environmental, Health, and Safety Service Hub of Kaiser Permanente.

When examining how mold was addressed in its facilities, Kaiser Permanente discovered an inconsistency. "When some facilities discovered mold, they ignored it or painted over it, while other facilities called in consultants and spent thousands of dollars to remove the mold. Both these extremes were unacceptable. Our goal was to create a standardized practice regarding mold management that would be used throughout the entire Kaiser organization," stated Havel.

Creating the Program

To create its mold management program, Kaiser looked for guidance from APIC and AIA as well the American Industrial Hygiene Association (AIHA), ACGIH, the United States Environmental Protection Agency (USEPA), and the Centers for Disease Control and Prevention (CDC). "We wanted to create evidence-based processes that brought standardized practice to our facilities, managed risk to our staff and patients appropriately, and controlled costs," said Havel. The program was created by a subcommittee of Kaiser's National Building Issues Steering Committee (NBISC). "The group sequestered itself in a conference room for three days and discussed concepts in the morning and wrote guidelines in the afternoon," states Havel. The result of these work sessions was a draft of Kaiser's national program on water intrusion and mold management (WIMM). This draft was reviewed, revised, and finalized based on input from key players throughout the organization.

Program Content

The WIMM program requires the creation of a midlevel management team that is charged with managing both water intrusion incidents and mold complaints in a facility. "This team helps ensure an appropriate response to water intrusion and mold issues that is consistent with organization policy," Havel said. Suggested members of the team include the facility manager or building engineer; an environmental services representative; an infection control professional; an environmental, health, and safety professional; a representative of capital projects (construction team); and a representative of union labor, among others. Depending on the type, size, and scope of the facility, the team members can vary.

The program also provides detailed guidelines and tools that the management team uses to conduct WIMM activities. One section of the program provides specific guidelines for properly responding to water intrusion incidents such as sewer backups, roof leaks, or pipe leaks. This section requires individuals who discover a water intrusion problem to report it to the management team. The section also addresses how the management team should assess the magnitude of the problem, manage the problem, and prevent the onset of mold. The document identifies three categories of potential water intrusion: clean water, gray water, and black water.

Chapter 2: Facility-Related Risks

Clean water intrusion occurs when uncontaminated water is released into the environment. This could occur when a drinking water supply line leaks or a sink, shower, or bath overflows. Rainwater entering a building through a roof, ceiling, or window is also considered a clean water intrusion. Gray water intrusion involves water that is used in equipment such as steam sterilizers and dishwashers. Any source of water emanating from equipment that does not contain or has not been contaminated by fecal matter is considered gray water. Black water contains or has been contaminated with fecal matter and includes toilet or sewer water. Each water type requires different responses and levels of protection for the response team. In addition, the program provides guidelines and standardized forms to help identify the patient populations potentially impacted by the water intrusion. The program designates different categories of response procedures based on the identified scope of the problem and patients affected. These responses can range from containing the water intrusion and drying it within 48 hours to evacuating areas contaminated by water and removing structural components such as walls that have been contaminated. After water is removed, the WIMM program recommends that the management team conduct a follow-up investigation including a visual inspection of the area, an interview with occupants of the area, and perceptions of unusual odors. The program recommends that the management team document the response effort and evaluate it for future improvement.

Another section of the WIMM program addresses managing the chronic issue of mold. The guidelines and tools found in this section come into play when a complaint is filed about the presence of mold. For example, if during a construction project a wall is taken down and mold is discovered, the WIMM program addresses how that mold issue should be handled. The response procedures are similar to those of water intrusion incidents. The WIMM program requires an assessment of mold severity and patient risk and the implementation of procedures that reflect the seriousness of the assessment. A follow-up investigation, documentation, and analysis are also recommended. "The mold management piece is linked to water intrusion management. Mold happens when a building system fails. If we focus only on removing the presence of mold, we address a symptom; we don't necessarily solve our problem. Mold grows where there is water, so an integral part of mold management is identifying where the water is and eliminating it. If there is no water, then there is no mold," Havel stated.

Implementing the Program

After the program was created, Kaiser spent time educating staff on the program. The organization conducted a teleconference that was simulcast to all Kaiser facilities. In addition, education is provided at monthly infection control meetings. "The program is still in flux, and we make changes to it as our facility staff provides feedback," said Havel.

To gauge the effectiveness of the WIMM program, Kaiser looks at those Kaiser facilities that have used the program to address a WIMM incident. "We look at how the WIMM program was implemented and the results of

---

Case at a Glance

Main Challenge: Develop a program that provides standardized response procedures and protocols addressing water intrusion incidents and mold management.

Issues: Lack of regulatory requirements on mold management that provide direction as to appropriate response. Varying levels of mold response efforts found throughout the organization.

Joint Commission Standards: EC.1.10, EC.1.20, EC.8.10, EC.9.10, EC.9.20, EC.9.30

Solutions: Developed a program based on guidance from national environment of care (EC) organizations and input from a multidisciplinary team. The program includes assessment and response guidelines based on the level of risk to the patient and employee. It also establishes a management-level response team to spearhead response efforts.

Outcomes: The organization has increased protection of staff and patients, standardized its approach to WIMM, and reduced its reliance on outside consultants to address water and mold issues.

the program," Havel said. "The program is designed so that organizations do not need to bring in a consultant to fix mold and water issues, except in the most extreme cases. One way of measuring the success of the program is to look at how many times a consultant is hired to manage a mold or water problem. Since the WIMM program was implemented, we have seen a drop in the use of consultants," Havel said.

Although mold growth can be a potential health hazard under certain conditions if not properly managed, currently there are no specific regulatory requirements that dictate how identified mold growth should be managed or remediated. Kaiser's program provides appropriate guidelines to promptly, effectively, and efficiently address mold issues, and other organizations are looking to adapt Kaiser's plan for their facilities.[14]

ASBESTOS

Asbestos is a term that refers to a group of fibrous minerals found in rock formations. Asbestos is valuable industrially because it has high tensile strength, flexibility, heat and chemical resistance, and good frictional properties. It was commonly used in building materials of the 1940–1970 eras.

Asbestos is dangerous because, with processing or other disturbance, it separates into very thin microscopic fibers. The fibers are inhaled into the body or orally ingested and become embedded in the tissues of the respiratory or digestive system, respectively. Diseases caused by asbestos are asbestosis, a scarring of the lung tissue similar to emphysema; lung cancer; gastrointestinal cancer; and mesothelioma, a cancer of the membranes covering the body organs.[15]

The Joint Commission addresses the issues surrounding asbestos in several standards. For example, EC.1.10 requires organizations to manage safety risks and asbestos would qualify as a safety risk. EC.3.10 requires organizations to identify hazardous materials used, stored, or generated in the organization. Asbestos fibers would fall into this category. In EP3 of this standard the Joint Commission addresses the handling, storing, and disposing of hazardous materials, which would cover an asbestos abatement program.

EC.8.30, EP2, EP3, and EP4 address the need for a pre-construction risk assessment for any project involving construction, renovation, and demolition. Evaluation of the area to be renovated or demolished should include an assessment for the presence of asbestos. If any is found, the organization should take action such as establishing an OSHA-compliant asbestos abatement program.

STANDARDS *Joint Commission Standards that Implicitly Address Asbestos*

▶ EC.1.10, Safety Management; EC.3.10, Hazardous Materials & Waste Management (EP3); EC.8.30, Built Environment (EP2, EP3, EP4)

Hazard Identification

It is important for health care organizations to keep records of the presence and quantity of any asbestos-containing material, or material presumed to contain asbestos, present in a building. OSHA has specific requirements regarding this issue including that records should be kept for the term of facility ownership and then be transferred to subsequent owners. In buildings built before 1980, thermal system insulation and sprayed-on or troweled-on surfacing materials should be presumed to contain asbestos unless analyzed to contain less than 1% asbestos. The same is true for asphalt and vinyl flooring installed before 1980. Asbestos may also be contained in the materials shown in Figure 2-1. Note that not every item that fits a description in this figure contains asbestos, nor is the figure inclusive.

Asbestos Exposure

OSHA has set specific permissible exposure limits (PELs) for asbestos. All projects that may involve asbestos must be evaluated to determine the potential to generate airborne asbestos fiber. If the airborne concentration may exceed the PEL, employees must be initially monitored for exposure within their breathing zone. If these measurements are above the limits, monitoring must be repeated at least every six months. However, if the initial monitoring was below the limits, monitoring for that project may be discontinued, unless a change occurs that may increase the exposure.

OSHA requires a written program to reduce exposure, if exposure has been determined to be an issue. Employee rotation may not be used to reduce the exposure. Employers must notify impacted employees of the results of monitoring and any corrective action

Figure 2-1. Materials That May Contain Asbestos[16]

Cement pipes	Elevator brake shoes
Cement wallboard	HVAC duct insulation
Cement siding	Boiler insulation
Asphalt floor tile	Breaching insulation
Vinyl floor tile	Ductwork flexible fabric connections
Vinyl sheet flooring	Cooling towers
Flooring backing	Pipe insulation
Construction mastics	Heating and electrical ducts
Acoustical plaster	Electrical panel partitions
Decorative plaster	Electrical cloth
Textured paints/coatings	Electric wiring insulation
Ceiling tiles and lay-in panels	Chalkboards
Spray-on insulation	Roofing shingles
Blown-in insulation	Roofing felt
Fireproofing materials	Base flashing
Taping compounds (thermal)	Thermal paper products
Packing materials for wall/floor penetrations	Fire doors
High-temperature gaskets	Caulking/putties
Laboratory hoods and table tops	Adhesives
Laboratory gloves	Wallboard
Fire blankets	Joint compounds
Fire curtains	Vinyl wall coverings
Elevator equipment panels	Spackling compounds

These are among the asbestos-containing materials found in a health care environment.
Source: U.S. Environmental Protection Agency.

being taken in writing, either via individual notification or by posting a notice. Exposure monitoring records must be kept for 30 years.

Medical Surveillance

OSHA mandates a program of medical surveillance for all employees who are exposed to asbestos at levels above the PEL. This involves a medical examination, available annually, and performed or supervised by a licensed physician, provided at no cost to the employee. Minimum components of this exam include, but are not limited to, medical and work history, complete physical exam emphasizing respiratory, cardiovascular, and digestive systems, chest X-ray, and pulmonary function tests. The employee must be notified of the results of this medical examination.

Regulated Areas

According to OSHA, any areas within a building where asbestos exposure exceeds or may exceed permissible exposure limits must be designated as regulated areas with entry restricted only to those who are authorized. Authorized entrants are required to wear a respirator. (See Chapter Three for information on respiratory protection.) Regulated areas must have posted signage at all entrances. The signs must be in languages that all employees can understand, and must use pictures if necessary. Asbestos products and waste containers must also be labeled.

Training

The Joint Commission emphasizes that all employees should be trained regarding the risks of their job responsibilities. These risks would include asbestos risks depending on the employee's job responsibility. OSHA also has requirements regarding asbestos training. As mentioned previously, the Joint Commission does not require compliance with these requirements, but they are provided here as food for thought. OSHA requires organizations to provide employees who are exposed to asbestos at concentrations at or above PELs with training upon their assignment to the area and at least annually thereafter. Content of the program should include information such as the effective ways to safeguard health; the relationship between smoking and exposure to asbestos in the development of lung cancer; the quantity, location, use, release, and storage of asbestos; the procedures to protect employees; and the nature of operations that could result in exposure.[17]

It is important to note that housekeepers in buildings that contain asbestos or asbestos-containing materials may also be exposed. According to OSHA, the housekeepers must receive awareness-level training, repeated at least annually. Once again, training must be presented in a language that is understandable to the employee.

Controls

Organizations can reduce employee exposure to asbestos in a variety of ways. For example, engineering and work practice controls can be used. OSHA's requirements regarding engineering and work practice controls are as follows:

- Use local exhaust ventilation and dust collection systems
- Use local exhaust ventilation for hand-operated and power tools that produce or release asbestos fibers
- Handle, mix, apply, remove, cut, score, or work asbestos when it is wet to prevent fiber release
- Do not remove asbestos-containing materials from shipping containers without wetting, enclosing, or ventilating them
- Do not sand floors containing asbestos
- Do not use compressed air to remove asbestos unless in conjunction with a ventilation system designed to collect the dust[15]

The use of PPE can also reduce employee exposure to asbestos. PPE should be used when the above controls are not able to reduce the exposure to appropriate levels. They should also be used as engineering controls are being installed, when engineering controls are not feasible, and during emergencies.

Organizations should provide protective clothing to the employee working where asbestos concentrations are high. This clothing includes full-body clothing, such as coveralls, head coverings, gloves, and foot coverings. Eye protection may be necessary if the possibility of eye irritation exists. According to OSHA, protective clothing must be removed in changing rooms and placed in closed labeled containers that prevent the release of asbestos fibers following work in a regulated area. Clean clothing must be provided at least weekly, and the associated hazards and controls must be communicated to those who launder these items. When being removed from changing rooms, contaminated clothing must be transported in sealed and labeled containers.

More information about OSHA's specific requirements regarding asbestos can be found on http://www.osha.gov.

HEARING CONSERVATION

Noise is unwanted sound. Sound is caused by pressure changes in the air from a vibrating source. Hearing loss may be caused by the exposure to high levels of noise, increasing with the duration of the exposure and the intensity of the noise.

Hearing loss resulting from noise exposure may be temporary with short-term exposures to noise. After a period away from the noise, normal hearing usually returns. A common example of this phenomenon is the temporary hearing loss experienced after attendance at a loud rock concert or dancing near an amplifier of a live band.

If exposure to noise is long term and the noise levels are high, permanent damage can result. Elevated noise levels may also lead to reduced productivity, decreased communication among staff members, and other physiological changes.[18]

The Joint Commission implicitly addresses the issue of noise exposure and hearing conservation under standard EC.1.10: the effective environmental management program for the safety of staff members and others.

STANDARDS *Joint Commission Standards that Implicitly Address Hearing Conservation*

➤ EC.1.10, Safety Management
➤ HR.2.10, Initial Job Training; HR.2.20, Roles & Responsibilities; HR.2.3, Ongoing Education

Figure 2-2. Permissible Noise Exposures[20]

DURATION PER DAY (HOURS)	SOUND LEVEL (dBA)
8	90
6	92
4	95
3	97
2	100
1.5	102
1	105
0.5	110
<0.25	115

OSHA mandates a hearing conservation program when sound exceeds these levels.

Source: U.S. Department of Labor, Occupational Safety and Health Administration.

Noise Levels and Monitoring

A decibel (dB) is a unit of relative sound intensity. On the decibel scale, 0 dB is the average least perceptible sound and 130 dB is the average pain level. This is a logarithmic scale, with sound doubling every 10 dB. The decibel time weighted average (TWA) is expressed as dBA.[18] The dBA scale is devised to respond to inputs of 40 dB.

OSHA has identified an eight-hour TWA action level for noise exposure of 85 dBA[†]. All employees who are exposed to noise at or above this action level must be part of a hearing conservation program. To measure the TWA, all "continuous, intermittent, and impulsive noise within an 80 dB to 130 dB range[19] must be measured in the normal work setting." If the work setting changes, monitoring must be repeated. Some employers choose to repeat monitoring periodically as a matter of course.

OSHA mandates a hearing conservation program not only based on the action level, but when sound levels exceed those shown in Figure 2-2.

Employees should be permitted to observe noise monitoring, and they must be informed of its outcomes. According to OSHA, noise exposure records must be kept for two years.

Only employers who suspect workplace noise to be in excess of 85 dBA need to conduct monitoring. Indications that this might be necessary are employee complaints about loud noise, indications of employee hearing loss, or conditions under which normal conversations are difficult. Areas in health care facilities that usually have elevated noise levels are the mechanical rooms, machine shops, garages, and the print shop. The food service department and the laboratory may also merit evaluation for noise levels.

Noise can be measured with a sound level meter or a dosimeter. A sound level meter measures sound intensity at a given moment, thus requiring multiple measurements at different times and locations within the given workplace to develop an estimate of exposure over a workday. If the levels change over the

---

† OSHA has several regulations related to occupational noise exposure, as follows:
29CFR 1910.95	Occupational noise exposure
Appendix A	Noise exposure computation
Appendix B	Methods for estimating the adequacy of hearing protector attenuation
Appendix C	Audiometric measuring instruments
Appendix D	Audiometric test rooms
Appendix E	Acoustic calibration of audiometers
Appendix F	Calculations and application of age corrections to audiograms
Appendix G	Monitoring noise levels nonmandatory informational appendix
Appendix H	Availability of referenced documents
Appendix I	Definitions
29CFR 1904	Recording and Reporting Occupational Injuries and Illnesses
1904.10	Recording criteria for cases involving occupational hearing loss
29CFR 1926.52	Occupational Noise Exposure

Much of the appendix material is technical information related to the audiometric measurements, and is beyond the scope of this document. Audiometric testing in general, however, will be discussed subsequently.

course of the day, the length of time at each noise level should also be determined.

A dosimeter stores the measurements of sound levels and integrates them over time to yield an average noise exposure. A microphone is placed near the employee's ear and it is read at the end of the day.[21]

Audiometric Testing

OSHA requires a program of audiometric testing by the employer to monitor the hearing of employees who are exposed to noise at or above the 85 dBA action level. Audiometric testing measures the employee's hearing level over time.

This program must be under the responsibility of a licensed or certified audiologist, otolaryngologist (ear, nose, throat specialist), or other physician. This physician may conduct the testing, or a qualified technician may conduct the testing without the physician present. The physician, however, must review all audiograms that reveal a problem and make appropriate recommendations for referral.

When doing audiometric testing, organizations should establish a baseline with each employee. Thereafter, annual audiograms are compared with the baseline to identify any hearing loss. Each test should be recorded including the employee's name, job classification, date of the test, examiner's name, results of the test, and so forth.

A standard threshold shift (STS) is used as the measure of hearing loss. This is an average shift in either ear of 10 dB or more at pitches of 2,000, 3,000, and 4,000 Hertz. Hertz (Hz) is a measure of frequency or pitch measured in cycles per second.[18] Any employee whose audiogram shows an STS (with hearing protectors in use during work) must have those protectors fit or refit. They must be trained or retrained in their use. This STS must be recorded on the OSHA 300 log. Employers must also record work-related hearing loss when the audiogram shows a marked decrease in overall hearing. This may be adjusted for aging.

Hearing Protection

Under OSHA's requirements, hearing protection must be provided to all employees who are exposed to the 85 dBA. A selection of at least one type of ear plug and one type of ear muff must be provided, and the employee may choose one that is comfortable and provides sufficient protection. A noise reduction rating is provided for each hearing protector to allow for appropriate selection.

If noise levels change in the workplace, the protectors may need to be changed to accommodate that. All hearing protectors used must reduce the noise to at least 90 dBA, and if an STS has already occurred, the noise level must be reduced to 85 dBA.

Any employees exposed to noise at or above the action level of 85dBA must participate in a training program at least annually. Topics to be covered in such a training program include the effects of noise; the purpose, advantages, and disadvantages of types of hearing protectors; and the purpose of and procedures for audiometric testing.

MACHINE GUARDING

Any use of machinery or equipment with moving parts can be a potential source of injury if a worker places a body part in harm's way. Loose clothing, hair, and jewelry can become entangled, accidentally drawing the worker into a dangerous position. Hands and arms may be crushed or severed, projectiles from equipment may cause blindness, and the list goes on.

Various types of motions in machinery or equipment can be hazardous. The potential for problems increases if any moving parts have projections. One source of hazards in machinery is nip points. Nip points are the points at which two parts of the machinery come together in a way that can be hazardous to the worker. These can be created by parts that are either in contact or close proximity rotating in opposite directions, such as intermeshing gears. Another type of nip point is created between rotating parts and others that move in a tangent to them, such as the point of contact between a belt and its pulley. Nip points may also be created between a part that moves back and forth and one that is stationary. Parts that move in a straight, continuous line over a stationary object may create hazards by catching a worker in a pinch or shear point.

In health care organizations, examples of the types of equipment, and their potential locations, that may be at risk for harming workers include the following:
- Radial arm saws: carpentry shops
- Lathes: carpentry shops
- Grinder: mechanical rooms, maintenance shops
- Emergency electrical generator: mechanical room
- Air handlers: various locations

Machine guards prevent access to moving parts that can cause injury, and therefore represent engineering controls to safety. Safeguards should be provided for any machine part or process that can cause injury. These fall into three general areas. The first is the

Chapter 2: Facility-Related Risks

point of operation of the machinery, such as cutting or boring. Second, parts of the mechanical system that transmit energy to the point of operation, such as pulleys, belts, connecting rods, and gears, are a potential hazard source. Finally, all other moving parts can cause injury if not guarded.

Standards and Regulations

The Joint Commission's requirement for effective management of an environmental health and safety program found in EC.1.10 governs the implementation and use of machine guards because these can help ensure employee safety.

STANDARDS — *Joint Commission Standards that Implicitly Address Machine Guarding*

► EC.1.10, Safety Management;
► HR.2.10, Initial Job Training; HR.2.20, Roles & Responsibilities; HR.2.30, Ongoing Education

---

OSHA has a number of regulations relating to machine guarding in general and others unique to particular industries. Because hospitals perform many functions typical to other industries, applications of the more specific regulations to certain activities within health care may be limited.[‡] While Joint Commission does not survey for compliance with OSHA regulations, those regulations are listed here for consideration.

For all types of equipment, OSHA requires one or more methods of machine guarding to protect the operator and other employees in the machine area from hazards.[22] If at all possible, the guard should be attached to the machine itself. If this is not possible, the guard may be secured elsewhere.

Any guarding that is put in place should prevent contact between the worker and the hazard. A guard must be secure (not easily removed or defeated) and must prevent any falling objects from entering the machine's moving parts. Guards should not introduce a new hazard into the system, nor should they interfere with the performance of work. If at all possible, guards should permit appropriate lubrication of the equipment without their removal. According to OSHA, "engineering controls that eliminate the hazard at the source and do not rely on the worker's behavior for their effectiveness offer the best and most reliable means of safeguarding."[23]

Safeguards

A variety of methods can be used to provide appropriate machine safeguards. Factors influencing the selection include the operation itself, the size and shape of the stock being used in the machine, the physical layout, and any requirements or limitations imposed by production needs. The safeguard chosen for the job should be the most effective and practical safeguard possible.

This discussion will focus on two classifications of these safeguards: guards and devices. Other possible safeguards are more unique to particular equipment, such as location/distance, feeding and ejection methods, and miscellaneous aids.

Guards

Guards are actual physical barriers. They may be fixed, interlocked, adjustable, or self adjusting. Fixed guards are not dependent on moving parts, and are usually the preferable means of protection. Interlocked guards have a trip mechanism that shuts off the machine's power to remove the hazard. The machine cannot be restarted until the guard is back in place, but replacing the guard should not automatically restart the machine. OSHA suggests that all removable guards be interlocked. Adjustable guards accommodate different sizes of stock. Self-adjusting guards automatically create an opening large enough to introduce the stock. Various types of guards and their advantages and disadvantages are shown in Figure 2-3.

[‡] The OSHA machine guarding regulations are as follows:
29CFR 1910 Subpart O	Machinery and Machine Guarding
29CFR 1910.211	Definitions
29CFR 1910.212	General requirements for all machines
29CFR 1910.213	Woodworking machinery
29CFR 1910.214	Cooperage machinery (reserved)
29CFR 1910.215	Abrasive wheel machinery
29CFR 1910.216	Mills and calendars in the rubber and plastics industries
29CFR 1910.217	Mechanical power presses
29CFR 1910.218	Forging machines
29CFR 1910.219	Mechanical power transmission apparatus

Figure 2-3. Types of Guards[24]

METHOD	SAFEGUARDING ACTION	ADVANTAGES	LIMITATIONS
Fixed	Provides a barrier.	Many specific applications In-plant construction possible Maximum protection Minimum maintenance High production, repetitive operations	Potential visibility interference Limited to specific operations Removal for adjustment & and repair
Interlocked	Shuts off or disengages power. Prevents starting when guard is removed.	Maximum protection Access for removing jams	Adjustment and maintenance May be easy to disengage jams
Adjustable	Provides a barrier that may be adjusted to suit operations.	Can suit specific operations Can be adjusted for varying sizes stock	Protection may not always be complete May need frequent maintenance and of adjustment
Self-Adjusting	Provides a barrier that moves with the size of the stock.	Commercially available	Does not always provide maximum protection Potential visibility interference May need frequent maintenance and adjustment

Various machine guards have different pros and cons.
Source: U.S. Department of Labor, Occupational Safety and Health Administration.

Devices

Devices perform specific functions to keep the worker from harm. They may be presence-sensing, pullback, or restraint types. Presence-sensing devices may stop a machine if a body part is placed in the danger area. They use photoelectric or radio frequency sensing devices that can interrupt the operating cycle of the machine if the light or capacitance field is broken. These devices may only be used if the machine can stop in time to prevent harm to the worker. Another type of presence-sensing device is electromechanical; these devices prevent the machine from starting if an object, such as a body part, prevents the device from attaining its proper position. Pullback devices are cables attached to the workers hands, wrists, or arms, and are applicable to machinery that uses a repeated stroking action. These devices permit the worker to access the operating area of the equipment only when it is safe to do so, and automatically withdraw the body parts when the machine stroke begins. Similarly, restraint devices use cables or straps attached to the operator to prohibit reaching into the hazardous area.

Guard Construction

According to OSHA requirements, it is permissible for guards to be designed and installed by the manufacturer of the equipment or by the user. The former tends to conform to the design and function of the machine, and may provide strengthening of the machine. User-built guards may be the only practical solution, particularly with older machinery, and can be customized to unique needs. But guards designed and built by the user may not conform to the machine configuration and function, and may not be properly designed or built.

Metal is often the best material for guards. Wood is usually not recommended because of poor durability and strength, and flammability. Wood guards are not prohibited by OSHA, however, and may be best for use with corrosive materials.

Ideally, routine lubrication and adjustment of the equipment should be possible without removal of the safeguards. Lockout/tagout mechanisms, described earlier in this chapter, would be an acceptable alternative.

Training

Workers using guarded machinery must understand what they are using and why. They must participate in training that is either instructional or hands-on. Topics should include the following:

- a description and identification of the hazards associated with particular machines

CHAPTER 2: FACILITY-RELATED RISKS

- The safeguards themselves, how they provide protection, and the hazards for which they are intended
- How to use the safeguards and why
- How and under what circumstances safeguards can be removed and by whom (in most cases repair or maintenance personnel only)
- What to do (for example, contact the supervisor) if a safeguard is damaged, missing, or unable to provide adequate protection.[23]

This training is extremely important because guards that have been removed or defeated provide no protection whatsoever. Workers must understand the importance of the guards and the necessity of leaving guards in place.

CONCLUSION

Both the Joint Commission and OSHA require organizations to identify and address those safety risks that are related to an organization's facilities. If an organization's facilities are harboring unseen and unidentified risks, they can significantly contribute to an unsafe work environment for staff. Appropriately addressing the risks found in an organization's facilities requires open communication among multiple disciplines, leadership support, employee participation, risk assessment, and education and training. ∎

References

1. U.S. Department of Labor: Occupational Safety and Health Administration: *Permit-Required Confined Spaces*. http://www.osha.gov/pls/oshaweb/owadisp.show_document?p_table=STANDARDS&p_id=9797 (accessed Mar. 19, 2005).

2. U.S. Department of Labor: Occupational Safety and Health Administration: *Fire Prevention Plans*. http://www.osha.gov/pls/oshaweb/owadisp.show_document?p_table=STANDARDS&p_id=12887 (accessed Mar. 19, 2005).

3. U.S. Department of Labor: Occupational Safety and Health Administration: *Coverage and Definitions*. http://www.osha.gov/pls/oshaweb/owadisp.show_document?p_table=STANDARDS&p_id=12886 (accessed Mar. 19, 2005).

4. U.S. Department of Labor: Occupational Safety and Health Administration: *General Requirements*. http://www.osha.gov/pls/oshaweb/owadisp.show_document?p_table=STANDARDS&p_id=9880 (accessed Mar. 19, 2005).

5. U.S. Department of Labor: Occupational Safety and Health Administration: *Control of Hazardous Energy (Lockout/Tagout)* 29CFR 1910.147. http://www.osha.gov/dts/osta/lototraining/tutorial/printer.htm (accessed Mar. 19, 2005).

6. Klingelsmith W.: *Indoor Air Quality: A Guide for Facility Managers*. American Society for Healthcare Engineering, 1995.

7. Baril G.: Indoor Air Quality – Investigation and Control. American Society for Healthcare Engineering Annual Conference, 1999.

8. Burroughs H. E. B.: IAQ: An Environmental Factor in the Indoor Habitat. *Heating/Piping/Air Conditioning* Feb. 1997.

9. Joint Commission Resources: *Infection Control Issues in the Environment of Care*, Oakbrook Terrace, IL: Joint Commission on Accreditation of Healthcare Organizations, 2004.

10. Joint Commission Resources: What Toronto hospitals learned from SARS. *Environment of Care® News* 7: 1-3 and 9, Jul. 2004.

11. Joint Commission Resources: *Environment of Care Handbook*. Oakbrook Terrace, IL: Joint Commission on Accreditation of Healthcare Organizations, 2004.

12. U.S. Department of Labor: Occupational Safety and Health Administration: *OSHA Technical Manual*. http://www.osha.gov/dts/osta/otm/otm_vi/otm_vi_1.html (accessed Mar. 19, 2005).

13. Hansen, W., et al: *A Guide to Managing Indoor Air Quality in Healthcare Organizations*. Oakbrook Terrace, IL: Joint Commission Resources, 1997.

14. Interview with Tim Havel, director of the Western Environmental, Health, and Safety Service Hub of Kaiser Permanente. Feb. 24, 2005.

15. U.S. Department of Labor: Occupational Safety and Health Administration: *Asbestos Standard for General Industry*. http://www.osha.gov/Publications/osha3095.pdf (accessed Mar. 19, 2005).

16. U.S. Environmental Protection Agency Region 6: *Asbestos-Containing Materials*. http://www.epa.gov/Region06/6pd/asbestos/asbmatl.htm (accessed Mar. 19, 2005).

17. U.S. Department of Labor: Occupational Safety and Health Administration: *Asbestos*. http://www.osha.gov/pls/oshaweb/owadisp.show_document?p_table=STANDARDS&p_id=9995 (accessed Mar. 19, 2005).

18. Tweedy J.T.: *Healthcare Hazard Control and Safety Management*. Boca Raton, FL: GR/St. Lucie Press, 1997.

19. U.S. Department of Labor: Occupational Safety and Health Administration: *Hearing Conservation*. http://www.osha.gov/Publications/osha3074.pdf (accessed Mar. 19, 2005).

20. U.S. Department of Labor: Occupational Safety and Health Administration: *Occupational Noise Exposure*. http://www.osha.gov/pls/oshaweb/owadisp.show_document?p_table=STANDARDS&p_id=10625&p_text_version=FALSE (accessed Mar. 19, 2005).

21. U.S. Department of Labor: Occupational Safety and Health Administration: *Monitoring Noise Levels Non-Mandatory Informational Appendix*. http://www.osha.gov/pls/oshaweb/owadisp.show_document?p_table=STANDARDS&p_id=9742 (accessed Mar. 19, 2005).

22. U.S. Department of Labor: Occupational Safety and Health Administration: *General Requirements for All Machines*. http://www.osha.gov/pls/oshaweb/owadisp.show_document?p_table=STANDARDS&p_id=9836 (accessed Mar. 19, 2005).

23. U.S. Department of Labor: Occupational Safety and Health Administration: *Basics of Machine Guarding*. http://www.osha.gov/Publications/Mach_SafeGuard/chapt1.html (accessed Mar. 19, 2005).

24. U.S. Department of Labor: Occupational Safety and Health Administration: *Methods of Machine Safeguarding*. http://www.osha.gov/Publications/Mach_SafeGuard/chapt2.html (accessed Mar. 19, 2005).

Chapter 3:

Human Factor-Related Risks

Many of the safety risks that organizations face in the workplace are the result of human behavior, rather than task-related issues. Other safety risks relate to personnel policies and procedures. This chapter will review some of the common risks related to both personnel and behavior including workplace violence prevention, ergonomics, emergency action planning, personal protective equipment (PPE), and respiratory protection. As in previous chapters, both Joint Commission and OSHA requirements are discussed. The Joint Commission does not require compliance with OSHA standards; OSHA requirements are discussed here as issues to consider when addressing worker safety concerns.

Violence Prevention in the Workplace

Workplace violence, as defined by the National Institute for Occupational Safety and Health (NIOSH), is "violent acts (including physical assaults and threats of assaults) directed toward persons at work or on duty."[1] Workplace violence can cover a variety of acts including verbal threats to inflict bodily harm, including vague or covert threats; attempting to cause physical harm by striking, pushing, and other aggressive physical acts; verbal harassment such as abusive or offensive language, gestures, or other discourteous conduct; disorderly conduct including shouting, throwing, or pushing objects, punching walls, and slamming doors; making false, malicious, or unfounded statements against another individual that tend to damage his or her reputation or undermine his or her authority; and even terrorism against workers. Figure 3-1 lists incidents that would fall into the category of workplace violence, but is not all-inclusive.

Acts of workplace violence may be grouped into three categories:
1. Violence by strangers
2. Violence by customers or clients
3. Violence by co-workers or by personal relations

In the workplace, violence is usually of a personal nature and is directed toward one individual or potentially against the organization as a whole. In a health care setting, the most common pattern of violence is care recipient against staff, followed closely by visitor against staff, and third, staff against care recipient.[2]

Figure 3-1. Examples of Workplace Violence

Beating	Psychological trauma
Stabbing	Threats or obscene phone calls
Suicide	Intimidation
Near suicide	Harassment of any kind
Shooting	Being followed
Rape	Being sworn or shouted at

Workplace violence can range from mild to extreme.

The workplace itself may be any location, either permanent or temporary, where an employee performs any work-related duty. This includes, but is not limited to, the buildings and the surrounding perimeters of an organization, field locations, and clients' homes. In addition, traveling to and from work assignments falls under the term workplace.

Violence can break out anywhere, at any time. For example, in one case a care recipient on a general medical unit flew into a rage, used a fire extinguisher to smash a room window, then took a large piece of glass from the window and approached another care recipient who was lying in bed. After unsuccessful attempts by hospital security officers and then police to convince the aggressor to put down the glass, including firing several nonlethal beanbag rounds to no effect, police officers shot and critically wounded the aggressor. In another case, a man whose mother died at hospital A, several months after undergoing a hip replacement at hospital B, brought a gun to hospital B, apparently targeting a nurse who had cared for his mother. Instead, he shot and killed the chief pharmacist, a nursing assistant, and the director of environmental services before being subdued by another visitor and a care recipient.[2]

Statistics

Homicide is the second-leading cause of death in the workplace in the United States. Statistics for 1997 show 856 workplace homicides, and nearly 2 million assaults and threats of violence. The economic impact of workplace violence is 1,175,100 lost workdays each year, representing 500,000 employees and $55 million in lost wages. When lost productivity, legal expenses, property damage, diminished public image, and increased security needs are considered, the national costs are in the billions of dollars.

Health care and social service workers are faced with a statistically significant rate of workplace violence. Between 1996 and 2000, there were 69 homicides in health services. In 2000, this sector contained 48% of all nonfatal injuries resulting from workplace assaults. The majority of these incidents took place in hospitals, nursing and personal care facilities, and residential care services.[3]

Risk Factors

Workplace violence in health care has a variety of risk factors. Following is a brief discussion of some of those risks.

Handguns

Handguns and other weapons are increasingly prevalent among patients, their families, and friends. To some extent, this may be geographically related, but not exclusively. During a four-year period in the late 1980s and early 1990s, researchers at Henry Ford Hospital Emergency Department in Detroit screened patients and visitors using a system of walk-through metal detectors placed at the entrances to the Emergency Department (ED). Approximately 3.5% of those screened were found to be carrying hazardous items, the overwhelming majority of them knives; however, nearly 600 guns were found. These figures would have increased significantly had the same security measures been in place for individuals served, visitors, and staff of the entire hospital complex.[2]

Gangs

The criminal justice system is increasingly using hospitals for criminal holds and the care of acutely disturbed, violent individuals. Also, gangs present a significant threat to many health care facilities. Once thought of as an exclusively inner-city problem,

Chapter 3: Human Factor-Related Risks

gangs today have spread throughout the country into suburbs and rural areas. Their often brazen behavior can intimidate staff, visitors, and care recipients alike. When a gang member is being treated in a facility for wounds suffered at the hands of a rival gang, the conflict often continues right into the ED, sometimes flowing to surgery and the intensive care unit. Even when warring factions gather only in the parking lot, serious confrontations affecting other people and property can take place. Hospitals have even experienced drive-by shootings into the entry and waiting areas of the ED.[2]

Mentally Ill Persons
Health care organizations are releasing an increasing number of acute and chronically mentally ill individuals without follow-up care. These individuals now have the right to refuse medication and can no longer be hospitalized involuntarily unless they pose a threat to themselves or others.

Treatment in the Home Setting
More and more medical treatment is being provided in the homes of patients, an environment over which the health care organization has little, if any, control. A home care environment poses a variety of risks not seen when care is provided within an organization's facilities. For example, home care workers may work alone in remote locations or high crime settings. See the following section on risk assessment for particular considerations for home care.

Temptations
Drugs and/or money are available at hospitals, clinics, pharmacies, and other health care organizations. This makes them a particular target for robbery. In most hospitals and clinics, the public has unrestricted movement. Joint Commission standard EC.2.10 EP6 calls for health care organizations to define their "security-sensitive" areas and control access and egress to them. Pharmacies and cash handling areas should be included in that listing. Another area usually designated as security-sensitive is the ED, for reasons of workplace violence prevention. The potential presence there of gang members, drug/alcohol abusers, trauma patients, and distraught family members increases the risk of violence.

Other risk factors for workplace violence include lower staffing levels during times of increased activity, such as meal and visiting times. Because many health care facilities work on a three-shift schedule, change of shifts that occur in the darkness may be subject to violence, particularly if the parking areas are poorly lit. Health care work is often isolated, such as work with clients during exams or treatment. Lack of training may result in failure to recognize and manage hostile and aggressive behavior.

Developing a Workplace Violence Prevention Program
Elements of a workplace violence prevention program can include the following:
- Effective leadership and employee involvement
- Worksite analysis
- Hazard prevention and control
- Training and education
- Recordkeeping and evaluation of the program

In some cases, development of a workplace violence prevention program may simply require linking various security and other policies and procedures already in place into a unified program. The resulting program must then be communicated to staff members for a clear understanding of the management support of this program.

STANDARDS *Joint Commission Standards that Address Workplace Violence*

➤ EC.1.10, Safety Management; EC.1.20, Environmental Tours; EC.2.10, Security Management (EP2, EP3, EP6); EC.4.10 Emergency Management (EP10); EC.9.10, Monitoring Environmental Conditions; EC.9.20, Analyzing Environmental Issues; EC.9.30, Improving the Environment
➤ HR.1.20, Qualifications (EP5); HR.2.10, Initial Job Training; HR.2.20, Roles & Responsibilities

---

Effective Leadership
For any safety and health program, management commitment is essential to its incorporation into the organizational culture and its ultimate success. Management must express the organizational concern for each employee's emotional and physical safety and health, demonstrating an interest at a level equal to that for the health and safety of patients and

their families. A system of accountability for both managers and employers should be established.

At the policy level, management must create and disseminate a clear policy of zero tolerance for workplace violence. This must include a means to ensure that no reprisals will be taken against employees who report incidents. Employees should be encouraged to promptly report incidents and to suggest ways to reduce or eliminate risks.

Management is responsible for a comprehensive security plan in the workplace. Joint Commission EC.2.10 EP2 requires an organization's leadership to designate a person or persons to coordinate the development, implementation, and monitoring of security management activities. Similarly, OSHA's guidelines* state that responsibility and authority be assigned to individuals with appropriate training and skills. And management communication to the employees should be ongoing.

Another important management practice that can contribute to the prevention of workplace violence is background screening for all applicants for employment. Joint Commission standard HR.1.20 EP5 calls for an organization to verify "information on criminal background" according to law, regulation, and organizational policy. Evidence suggest that, nationwide, between 25% - 40% of job applicants falsify their resumes. This is especially troubling to health care organizations of all kinds because employers can be held liable if their failure to adequately check on applicants' backgrounds results in harm to other employees or the public. Few members of the public are as vulnerable as individuals being served in health care organizations. Unfortunately, when these individuals are victims of violence, it is most often at the hands of staff.[2]

Employee Involvement

Under a workplace violence prevention program, employees are obligated to understand and comply with the program and associated safety and security measures. They should participate in available complaint and suggestion procedures and promptly report any incidents of violence. Other avenues for employee involvement would include participation on committees or teams that review incident reports and participation in continuing education programs on workplace violence prevention.

Each employee should be aware of and follow basic security expectations that have been taught in orientation and education programs. Some of those expectations particularly related to workplace violence prevention are shown in Figure 3-2.

Worksite Analysis

Part of any security risk assessment should include a worksite analysis, a systematic look at the workplace to find existing or potential hazards for workplace violence. This may be accomplished by assigning a team to evaluate areas of vulnerability throughout the organization and determine appropriate actions. This team's activities should include:

- Analyzing and tracking records

Sidebar 3-1. Workplace Violence in Home Care Settings

Home care settings pose particular risks for workplace violence, unusual to an institutionalized health care setting. When developing a workplace violence prevention program for home care, organizations should consider the following issues:

- Communication: Consideration should be given to providing the caregivers with communication devices, such as cellular telephones, so that they can quickly summon help if necessary.

- Area/Clientele served: A security risk assessment should evaluate particular risks for the area into which caregivers are traveling to visit clients. For example, crime rates should be evaluated. As a result of these assessments, an organization may determine that security or police escorts may be desirable for employees.

- Caregiver staffing: As a result of the risk assessment, it may be prudent to assign caregivers in pairs rather than sending them on solo assignments.

- Weapons: Will the caregivers be assigned to carry a weapon of any sort, such as pepper spray? If so, appropriate training must be provided.

- Domestic violence: One aspect of security training for home care providers should address the potential for the caregiver to walk into a situation of domestic violence, and his or her response to that situation.

- Dogs: Although many dogs are very friendly, dog bites are a statistically significant source of workplace injury. Home care providers should be provided with training to address this potential hazard.

---

* Due to the risk level of workplace violence in health care organizations, in 1996 OSHA Document 3148, "Guidelines for Preventing Workplace Violence for Health Care and Social Service Workers," first became effective. This document is not a regulation. It is advisory in nature and informational in content. The intent is that it be used by employers who are working to provide a safe and healthful workplace through effective workplace violence prevention programs.

Figure 3-2. Basic Security Expectations of Each Employee[2]

Employees can contribute to their own safety and security by taking the following steps:
- Use only assigned parking areas
- Enter and leave the facility only via assigned staff entrances
- Wear/display employee identification badge as and how required
- Question all strangers: "Can I help you?"
- Report suspicious activity relative to visitors, other staff, or care recipients
- Properly store and secure facility and personal property as per policy
- Never loan or duplicate issued keys
- Fully cooperate in any investigation or drug testing and comply with all facility policies and procedures

Employees can take a proactive stance toward ensuring their own security.

Source: Joint Commission Resources.

- Monitoring trends and analyzing incidents
- Screening employee surveys
- Analyzing workplace security

Joint Commission expects that workplace violence is one of the considerations made in an organization's proactive security risk assessment required by EC.2.10 EP3. Each health care organization must examine its security risks to determine which risks should be managed based on their probability of occurrence and impact to the organization. Conducting a risk assessment allows the organization to define those issues that pose a particular risk to the organization and therefore define the program and its boundaries.

TIP▶ Risk assessment for security should be based on a thorough evaluation of the facility and its grounds, the services offered, and the individuals served, as well as an examination of incident data and local crime statistics. This evaluation will undoubtedly include a review of employee health statistics, occurrence reports, and perhaps even safety reports to arrive at an estimation of the level of risk.[4] When reviewing security incidents, those that occur most frequently will probably be considered significant security risks. An annual review of area crime statistics with the local police department is prudent because any criminal activity that occurs in the community will not likely stop at the boundaries of the health care organization.

It is helpful to periodically have the security status reviewed by someone outside the organization so that a "fresh set of eyes" can pick up issues that might be missed by overly familiar staff members. This outside review may be accomplished by trading security officers with another organization or hiring an outside consultant.

Security risk assessment data is subject to change with time and should be reevaluated periodically.

Hazard Prevention and Control

After the workplace hazards have been identified, various means of hazard prevention and control should be implemented. These would include various types of controls, such as engineering controls to adapt the workplace, as well as administrative and work practice controls. A process should be established for post-incident response.

The OSHA workplace violence guideline provides numerous suggestions of controls that may be implemented. While these controls are not required by the Joint Commission, they can be helpful in preventing workplace violence. See Figure 3-3 for examples of various types of controls.

A number of these controls can be put into practice when designing an ED. See Sidebar 3-2 for a discussion of a security-focused design process.

TIP▶ One type of administrative control commonly used in health care organizations is a response team for situations involving violence or potential violence. Because many workers in health care settings are female, they may need to summon the physical strength of male employees on an urgent basis. Often there is an emergency code, such as "Mr. Strong," or a general workplace violence

Figure 3-3. Suggested Workplace Violence Controls

ENGINEERING CONTROLS	ADMINISTRATIVE AND WORK PRACTICE CONTROLS
Alarm systems	Zero tolerance policy
Metal detectors	Policy to report all incidents
Closed-circuit video	Management support during emergencies
Deep service counters	Trained response team
Bullet-resistant glass	Appropriate training of security officers
Curved mirrors	Controlled access, where appropriate
Waiting areas designed to minimize stress	Prohibition of working alone in emergency areas
Two exits for counseling or patient care rooms	Identification badges
Appropriate furniture arrangements	Security escorts to parking areas
Door locks	Visitation limitations as appropriate
Lighting	Home health policies and procedures

Workplace violence may be deferred by implementing these suggested control measures.
Source: U.S. Department of Labor, Occupational Safety and Heath Administration.

---

code, such as "Code Gray," to obtain that help. Appropriate training must be provided to designated responders to such a code.

TIP ▶ Occasionally, employees or patients in a health care organization will have a restraining order against another individual. It is prudent for management to have a policy that notification will be made to the organization in such an instance. Clearly privacy concerns surround this issue, but it is important for key individuals in the organization, such as the security staff, to be aware of these restraining orders and the identity of the individual named therein so that appropriate action can be taken if the individual comes to the organization with the intent to victimize the holder of the order.

If an incident of workplace violence does occur, leadership of the organization should, as a matter of policy, provide comprehensive treatment for any employees who have been victimized or traumatized by witnessing an incident of workplace violence. Included among the potential responses are trauma/crisis counseling, critical incident stress debriefing (CISD), and employee assistance programs to provide counseling and other assistance to the victims. The Joint Commission standard EC.4.10 EP10 addresses staff support activities in emergency situations. CISD is included as one of the items that must be provided by the health care organization to support staff members during or following an emergency, which would include a workplace violence incident.

Training and Education
All staff members should be aware of potential security hazards and ways of protecting themselves. All employees are potentially victims of workplace violence; therefore, training should involve all employees, including supervisors and managers. As part of the training program, employees should understand the concept of "Universal Precautions for Violence," that is, that violence should be expected but can be avoided or mitigated through preparation. Employees should be instructed to limit physical interventions in workplace altercations unless they have been specifically trained as part of a designated emergency response team.
- Suggested components of a training program include, but are not limited to:
- Workplace violence prevention policy
- Risk factors that cause or contribute to assaults
- Early recognition of escalating behavior or warning signs
- Ways to prevent volatile situations
- Standard response plan for violent situations
- Location and operation of safety devices

Figure 3-4 provides a listing of some of the safety devices frequently used in various departments that require specific training.

Chapter 3: Human Factor-Related Risks

One type of specific training that may be provided to individuals in selected positions is nonviolent crisis intervention. One of the primary features of such training is recognizing signs of escalating behavior. These signs are included in Figure 3-5, and could be exhibited by staff, visitors, or patients.

TIP ▶ Standard de-escalation techniques can be taught by in-house staff or an outside vendor. Good candidates for this training include staff members who are involved in situations in which anger is most apt to occur, such as staff working in behavioral health settings, EDs, admissions, and clinics; and support personnel such as security officers. Those individuals working in human resources or administration might also be potential candidates.

Trainees should regularly practice the techniques, using role playing, and take periodic refresher courses to maintain their competency in dealing with difficult situations. Figure 3-6 shows some of the basic elements of de-escalation training and ways to avoid certain practices that may be provocative.[2]

Recordkeeping

Recordkeeping and evaluation of the violence prevention program are necessary to determine the overall effectiveness of the program and to identify deficiencies or changes that should be made to the program. The OSHA 300 log (see Chapter Two) should be used to record medical reports of workplace injuries resulting from assaults. Organizations should record other information including the following:

- Incidents of abuse, verbal attacks, or aggressive behavior
- Patients with a history of violence
- Minutes of the safety committee
- Records of hazard analysis
- Corrective actions
- Training programs

Safety committee minutes can be especially telling. For example, review of one inpatient behavioral health organization's minutes revealed monthly reports of staff members being struck by patients—clearly an ongoing workplace violence problem in that these were not isolated incidents. The appropriate response might have included addressing the reasons for violence from a clinical perspective and/or training the staff members to de-escalate potentially violent situations.

Sidebar 3-2. Designing an Emergency Department for Safety

The ED. Is any area of a health care organization more ripe for violence? Care recipients arrive in acute physical and/or psychological distress, and the nature of emergency medicine demands fast-paced assessment, treatment, and disposition of the care recipient. To minimize the potential for violent behavior, health care organizations need to tightly control access to each of the four major areas of the ED: waiting, triage, treatment, and seclusion.

Waiting Area. As a reception area for ambulatory care recipients and a general waiting location, the waiting area can accommodate relatively free access. In some smaller facilities that have minimal staff, the entry could be locked but readily opened for arriving persons; use of a night bell, remote unlocking, and voice communication devices are common. Even in larger facilities where the entry point is open 24 hours per day, locking hardware would make it possible, should circumstances warrant, to quickly impose a total lockdown of the ED. The admissions function usually occupies space in the waiting area, and an admissions clerk is often the first person approached when the triage area or signs pointing to it are not readily apparent. To protect the admissions clerk from being grabbed or struck, a facility can enclose or semi-enclose the desk area. If this area does not open directly to the treatment area, it should be locked.

Triage Area. The triage area should be configured in much the same manner as the admissions desk area, with the exception that a patient must be able to easily access the triage area. Triage should open directly into the treatment area.

Treatment Area. Approximately half of all violent acts that occur in the ED take place in the treatment area. Good security practice dictates that all entry points to this area be locked, including those to the waiting room, x-ray, and laboratories. Either card access or push button locks can allow for staff entry.

Seclusion Room. Large EDs usually have dedicated seclusion rooms; smaller EDs often have rooms that can quickly be converted for this purpose. A seclusion room must allow for unhindered observation of care recipients. Because it will be free of any equipment and designed for care recipient safety, it may also be used as a police prisoner holding area.

Other Security Features. Organizations may want to consider using a closed-circuit TV security system in the ED for surveillance and control of the ambulance entry area (internal and external); for monitoring the waiting area and certain holding areas; and for care recipient observation in the seclusion room.

Walk-through metal detectors are used less frequently than closed-circuit TV systems. In general, the extremely high staffing cost and logistical problems of operating a viable comprehensive metal screening program in a medical facility do not make it cost effective for the ED. However, the use of a handheld metal detector can provide spot screening capability for situations that suggest a weapon may be present. Panic buttons are used by many EDs in remote treatment rooms, admissions areas, and triage areas. As with any other security device, periodic testing is essential to make panic buttons effective. Staff training and specific response protocols need to be current and comprehensive.[5]

■ ■ ■ Figure 3-4. Safety Devices Requiring Staff Training[2]

The following are examples of settings and devices that will require staff training:
- Laboratory: Late night access controls when limited staff are on duty
- Behavioral health: Unit-based closed circuit television
- Long-term care and assisted living: Ingress/egress exit alarm activation, resetting, and monitoring
- Emergency services: Panic alarm devices sending help signals to department or security facility locations
- Ambulatory care: Fire exit alarm and intrusion alarm systems
- Pharmacy: Panic/holdup alarms, access controls, vaults, and protected service counters

Source: Joint Commission Resources.

■ ■ ■ Figure 3-5. Signs of Confrontation and Escalating Negative Behavior[2]

The following behaviors and signals may indicate that confrontation is about to occur:
- Demanding unnecessary services or attention
- Acting chronically disgruntled
- Pacing with a display of being tense and angry
- Making unwarranted claims of entitlement
- Challenging authority
- Invading personal space
- Flushed face, twitching face or lips, and shallow breathing
- Escalating loudness, often with profanity
- Using overly aggressive actions and language, possibly due to intoxication or drug abuse
- Making statements about losing control (veiled threats)
- Opening and closing of the hands and/or using the index finger to point
- Darting or jerking eye movements, rapid looking around

Source: Joint Commission Resources.

TIP ▶ *Program Evaluation.*

As with all programs in a health care organization, the workplace violence prevention program should be in a state of continuous improvement. To maintain that, a uniform violence reporting system should be established, with a regular review of the reports. A review of safety committee minutes may also yield useful information (see previous paragraph). Employee health reports should be analyzed to look for trends in illness or injury caused by violence. Improvement in the program can be measured based on lowering the frequency and severity of workplace violence incidents. This is a potential security performance monitor for organizations that have an ongoing issue with workplace violence (see Chapter Five).

Violence prevention programs require support from leadership, participation from staff, risk analysis and control, and effective training and education. An example of how one organization developed its violence prevention program can be found on page 57.

Chapter 3: Human Factor-Related Risks

▪ ▪ ▪ Figure 3-6. Basic De-escalation Techniques in Managing Negative Behavior[2]

To de-escalate a situation, it is wise to do the following:

- Stand at an angle to the disturbed person, which is less threatening than directly facing him or her
- Do not invade personal space; stay at least four feet from the individual
- Do not maintain a rigid stance or cause the individual to feel cornered
- Do not touch the individual, unless it is necessary to manage extreme behavior
- Break eye contact with the individual to reduce the suggestion of aggression or control
- Ask the individual, "Why are you so angry?"
- Show that you are listening to the individual and respect his or her feelings
- Indicate that you want to help resolve the situation and do not make any promises you cannot keep
- Display sincerity, do not make threats, and do not set limits that you cannot enforce
- Clarify communication and ask for specific responses
- Ignore challenges and comment only on the person's behavior
- Move and speak slowly, quietly, and confidently

Source: Joint Commission Resources.

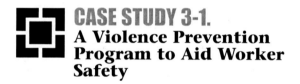

CASE STUDY 3-1.
A Violence Prevention Program to Aid Worker Safety

How the Veterans Health Administration Addresses Risks of Patient Violence to Workers in Multiple Health Care Settings

Imagine yourself as a physician, nurse, or other health care worker who's in training at a veterans administration hospital where you're focused on helping a patient with his health issues. Abruptly he breaks off his conversation with you, and as he comes at you, you see the glint of a knife in his hand.

This was the experience of Michael Hodgson, M.D., M.P.H, who now directs the Occupational Health Program at the Office of Environmental Health & Environmental Hazards at the Veterans Health Administration (VHA) in Washington, D.C. "Some providers assume that [violence] is part of being in health care," he said. "Many health care workers have had this kind of experience but think they're the exception." According to Hodgson, multiple surveys suggest that 11% - 12% of health care workers in the nation's 172 VHA facilities are the victims of patient assaults—the highest rate except for police and law enforcement officers.

Statistics show that, although they comprise less than 15% of the workforce in the United States, health care workers experience more than half of all the country's assaults.[6] Mental-health workers had a four-fold risk and registered nurses had an almost two-fold risk of assaults.[7] About 85% of the assaults at VHA facilities result from interactions with patients.

First Step: Create a Taskforce

In 2000, the VHA formed a National Taskforce on Violence Prevention, which included representatives from various VHA units and divisions. "Our first year was spent assessing violence in VHA and coming up with recommendations on how to prevent it," recalled Linda Belton, the taskforce co-chair and network director of one of 21 networks, that is, regional corporations, within VHA. The multidisciplinary taskforce included research specialists, representatives of labor organizations, and field personnel who are on the frontlines of patient care in health care facilities, especially those in nursing, emergency medicine, geriatrics, behavioral health, and rehabilitation.

Group members focused on several initiatives they considered vital to reducing patient assaults. First was the need among health care workers to stay alert to what was going on around them so they could predict and prevent violence. To that end, group members produced a 10-minute video designed to heighten awareness of violence. This video was shown during a specially designated time-out during which more than 90% of VHA employees participated in a one-hour awareness training session. The video is mandatory for all VHA personnel and is usually viewed by employees in groups where discussions are led by a trainer.

The group also designed a curriculum around Prevention and Management of Disruptive Behavior (PMDB), a program that has evolved since 1980. Employee training was strengthened, and the group identified high-risk groups to justify the high cost of training. "We started by training workers in high-risk groups, including emergency medicine, mental health, and geriatrics," said Belton. Each facility has two trainers to deliver the hands-on training needed to develop personal safety skills and de-escalation tactics, such as how to avoid challenging, insulting, or provoking the patient.

Leadership Commitment

The second initiative emphasized that VHA leadership is totally committed to protecting and supporting its staff. To strengthen and empower each facility's safety committee, those committees were expanded beyond engineering personnel to include clinical professionals and security specialists. Members of these safety committees began participating in safety rounds, in which leadership personnel at each VHA facility does a walk-around to identify safety issues. In addition to inspecting physical and structural safety factors, facility leaders query unit workers about their most recent training in violence prevention. The facility leaders also review the minutes of the safety committee and review the most recent results of workplace evaluations by the Joint Commission and other evaluators.

Facility leaders are also rated according to their performance in key aspects of violence prevention, including training members in high-risk groups, recruiting members for the local safety committees, and implementing a *flagging procedure*.

In August 2003 the VHA issued a directive requiring the systemwide use of Patient Record Flags (PRF). These flags alert VHA employees to patients whose behavior or characteristics may pose a threat to the safety of staff members and/or other patients, or might compromise quality health care delivery. Patients most likely to be flagged include those who have the following:

- A history of physical violence against patients or staff at a medical center or clinic
- Committed documented acts of repeated violence against others
- Made credible verbal threats of harm against specific individuals, patients, staff, or VA property
- Had possession of weapons or objects used as weapons in a health care facility
- A history of suicidal or parasuicidal behavior within health care facilities
- A history of repeated nuisance and disruptive or larcenous behavior that disrupts the environment of care
- A history of sexual harassment toward patients or staff

To help preserve a patient's right to treatment, members of a dedicated disruptive behavior committee under senior clinical leadership manage the use of PRF and review treatment. David Drummond, M.D., is a threat specialist who also manages the Mental Health Clinics at the VA Medical Center in Portland, Oregon. He recommends not adopting a punitive attitude toward a disruptive or violent patient. "It's understandable for someone to be angry when they've been threatened by someone who then has to be escorted out of the facility." He reminds his co-workers that federal law doesn't allow them to ban a disruptive patient from getting emergency care. "Our mission is to care for all eligible veterans," he said, "even those with a potential for violence."

In addition to the PRF, local computer software developed by the VHA is designed to alert health care workers about newly arriving patients who pose a high risk of violence. "An on-screen pop-up signals the presence of a high-risk patient and urges workers to put VA security staff on stand-by," said Drummond. "We studied a group of 50 high-risk patients for 12 months. We found that these Patient Record Flags virtually eliminated violence among this high-risk-for-violence patient group. We were able to set limits with them, get them examined, and care for them, and no one got hurt." Drummond and his colleagues found that the quality of health care for this group actually improved as a result of the limit-setting that the PRF put into motion.

The goal of the VHA is to prevent patient assaults by using a systematic approach to violence and creating a culture of safety. One component is to eliminate underreporting of violence. "We want to overcome any reluctance to reporting and have our employees feel comfortable about reporting incidents," Belton said. "We use an approach to reporting based on a model pioneered by NASA, in which employees are encouraged to report even a near-miss, where something could have occurred but didn't." In many cases, employees are acknowledged right on the spot. "Our facility directors celebrate anyone who brings forward a near-miss," she said. "It's only one of several areas where we're creating a whole culture of safety."

Recommendations

Hodgson, Drummond, and Belton have several recommendations for any organization that is concerned about reducing patient assaults. Among them are the following:

- Acknowledge where the patient is and explain what behavior is acceptable and what isn't
- Instead of penalizing workers for coming forward with information about safety, look for ways to support and reward reporting; encourage them to be part of finding a solution
- Because de-escalation skills are essential for health care workers, workers should get the tools they need to stay alert, pick up cues, defuse a situation, and handle violence if it erupts
- Establish and train a multidisciplinary violence risk assessment and threat management team
- Let workers know they have support and encouragement from the top on down

The taskforce also stresses that organizations should make it easy and painless for workers to speak up when they're frightened about the potential for violence from patients. "The natural impulse is to deny any concern in the hope it will go away," said Drummond. "I try to phone someone who's just been threatened or assaulted to ask if they're okay or to thank them for reporting an incident."

When an employee has suffered violence at the hands of a patient or another employee, Drummond recommends sitting down and debriefing that person in a confidential environment. "First, it's the humanitarian thing to do," he said. "And from a practical point of view, it's a good risk-management tool."

Hodgson adds that some patients may need special support for care, such as referring them to facilities where police officers are available.

"The survey, the Patient Record Flags, the training and retraining, the reporting methodology flags, and other safety measures we've instituted—all these are designed to provide a safe work environment for VHA employees," said Hodgson. "Furthermore, they're helping us ensure the right of all patients to receive health care that's confidential, safe and appropriate." [8]

The Program at a Glance

Main Challenge: Design, implement, and monitor a comprehensive program of violence prevention and protection for all workers in the Veterans Health Administration (VHA), the largest integrated health system in North America.

Issues: A taskforce reviewed violence within VHA, identified policy weaknesses and potential solutions, and made recommendations that included conducting a national survey.

Joint Commission Standards: EC.1.10. The health care organization manages safety risks. **EC.1.10 EP 5.** The health care organization uses the risks identified to select and implement procedures and controls to achieve the lowest potential for adverse impact on the safety and health of staff. **EC.2.10.** The health care organization identifies and manages its security risks. Rationale for **EC.2.10.** It is essential that a health care organization manages the personal security of staff.

Solutions: Survey workers, improve training, use computer alerts, implement an electronic flagging system in medical records to warn of high-risk patients, institute committees at each facility (under senior clinical leadership) to review assaults and recommend actions, flag management, heighten awareness and reward reporting actual incidents and near-misses.

Outcome: The VHA is working to reduce patient assaults through changing infrastructure, mandating training, creating a culture of safety, and promoting a culture of civility, respect, and patient empowerment.

Ergonomics

The science of ergonomics seeks to reduce the occurrence of musculoskeletal disorders (MSDs) by ensuring that each job is designed to accommodate the worker. An MSD is a disorder of the muscles, nerves, tendons, ligaments, joints, cartilage, blood vessels, or spinal disks caused by exposure to repetition, force, awkward postures, contact stress, and/or vibration to the back, neck, shoulder, elbow, hand, wrist, hip, knee, or ankle. Ergonomics considers human behavior, human characteristics and environmental conditions, along with the required job functions of an employee to develop a job and associated equipment that are a good fit to the worker.

The causes of MSDs are known as *ergonomic stressors*. Those that are particularly applicable to the health care industry are defined by OSHA as follows:

- Force: "The amount of physical effort required to perform a task (such as heavy lifting) or to maintain control of equipment or tools."
- Repetition: "Performing the same motion or series of motions continually or frequently."
- Awkward postures: "Assuming positions that place stress on the body, such as reaching above shoulder height, kneeling, squatting, leaning over a bed, or twisting the torso while lifting."[9]

Workers in health care organizations are prime candidates for MSDs. A frequent source is the lifting and/or repositioning of patients or residents, but there are others as well. A few examples would include pushing wheelchairs or gurneys, working in cold temperatures (such as operating rooms), prolonged computer use without support for the arms or legs, and various lifting and lowering actions such as lifting bags of laundry or trash, or as in storeroom work.

Statistics

Although the overall rate of occupational injuries has been trending down since 1992, the back injury rate for health care workers involved in direct patient care remains high. In fact, direct caregivers are still one of the most at-risk occupations. For years it was assumed that lifting patients was the major source of back injury problems in health care settings. However, this is belied by the results of a study that Guy Fragala, Ph.D., conducted when he was the director of environmental health and safety at the University of Massachusetts Medical Center in Worcester, Massachusetts. Working with Livia Pontani Bailey, R.N., B.S., M.A., risk control supervisor of the PMA Insurance Group in West Conshohocken, Pennsylvania, Fragala found that the major culprit in back injuries among health care employees was not lifting but repositioning patients.

To examine the problem of back injuries among health care workers, Fragala and Bailey first looked at figures from the Bureau of Labor Statistics (BLS) for 1998. Those data confirmed that 44% of work-related injuries were strains and sprains, mostly involving back injuries. Nearly 11% were caused by moving and helping patients in health care facilities.

The BLS stats further show that the occupations leading the injured list include nursing aides, orderlies, and attendants, with registered nurses not far behind. Government figures show that 66% of all injuries suffered by nursing aides and orderlies were strains and sprains, and 59% of all injuries suffered by registered nurses were strains and sprains.[7] In fact, the incidence rates calculated for overexertion as the cause for injuries in nursing and personal care facilities are four times higher than the national average for all industries.

Costs

Good ergonomics is good economics. The direct costs of occupational injuries include the expense of medical care and the compensation paid to injured workers—costs that are often covered by insurance. But health care organizations themselves must pay for the indirect costs related to occupational injuries. These can include replacing injured workers, additional training time by supervisors and administrators, loss of productivity, lowered morale, and other related issues.

The problem of back injuries is a major drain not just on health care budgets but also on the physical and emotional well-being of patient-care personnel. The nursing workforce is growing older, and experts predict critical shortages for the future. Within the next 10 years, the average age of a registered nurse will rise to more than 45 years, and 40% of the workforce will be more than 50 years old. Studies show that physical strength for most people begins to wane by age 40 and continues to drop as they approach age 50. This means that an older nursing force will be shouldering—literally—the physical demands of caring for dependent patients.[10]

Figure 3-7 identifies some factors in the work environment and their potential outcome in human and workplace costs, which ultimately translate to financial impacts for an organization.

Figure 3-7. Ergonomics and Musculoskeletal Disorders

WORK ENVIRONMENT FACTOR	POTENTIAL OUTCOMES
Work-related permanent disability	Lost time, medical costs, treatment costs, replacement costs, case management, low morale
Work-related temporary disability	Lost time, medical costs, replacement costs, investigation costs, case management
Work-related pain	Errors, performance decrease, employee turnover
Work-related discomfort	Errors, performance decrease, absenteeism
Poorly designed job	Errors, poor performance

Poor ergonomics can translate to negative financial effects.

Figure 3-8. Top Back-Injury Causes

1. Repositioning patients in bed (17%-18% of all occupational strains and sprains)
2. Lifting an object
3. Lifting a patient
4. Transferring a patient between bed and chair
5. Transporting a patient

Patient handling issues accounted for four out of the five top back-injury causes.

Problem Identification

To understand the nature of the problem facing health care organizations from back injuries in particular, it is important to identify which activities contribute to the highest injury rates. In their previously described study, Fragala and his colleague reviewed occupational injury experience from seven hospitals in the northeast portion of the United States over a period of two years. The hospitals ranged in size from 150 beds to 600 beds. Fragala analyzed the injury reports submitted to the workers' compensation carriers to determine which patient care activities were most involved in occupational strains and sprains.

His scrutiny revealed that four of the top five activities involved in injury causation at these seven hospitals were related to patient handling tasks, as shown in Figure 3-8.

In the past, health care organizations have attempted to resolve the problem of back injuries by teaching proper lifting technique. But multiple studies have demonstrated that this approach simply doesn't work for a variety of reasons including the following:

- Encouraging proper lifting techniques involves behavior modification, which seldom works on a long-term basis. Most workers revert to old behavior styles.
- Most training involves theory and is done in a classroom setting. But when workers move into the patient care environment, it is often difficult to apply theoretical principles.
- Because people are so different, no optimum principles apply universally to all workers. With the wide variety of possible situations, it is difficult to prescribe a single effective technique.

The techniques for moving and repositioning patients are founded on the principles for lifting objects. But patients and residents are not as compact as objects, less predictable than objects, and generally heavier than many objects. "Most workers can be trained in the proper way to lift an object such as a box," said Fragala. "But not only is that object more compact than a human being, it's more predictable. It doesn't do something unexpected as you're lifting it, the way patients can. And workers in a health care setting are always reaching out, which puts extra strain on their backs." [10]

Standards and Regulations

The Joint Commission addresses the issues of ergonomics in several parts of the Environment of Care (EC) standards. Organizations are encouraged to incorporate an ergonomics program under the umbrella of environmental health and safety. For example, as previously mentioned, EC.1.10 EP1 requires organizations to "effectively manage the environmental safety of patients, staff, and other people coming to the organization's facilities." Ergonomics is one aspect of environmental safety. A comprehensive, proactive risk assessment is required by EC.1.10 EP4. In examining the risks in a health care organization, the potential hazards for musculoskeletal disorders cannot be overlooked. After being identified, EC.1.10 EP6 states, "The organization establishes safety policies and procedures that are distributed, practiced, and reviewed." These three elements of performance form a logical sequence: provide for the safety by first identifying the risks and then implementing policies and procedures to appropriately manage the risks.

STANDARDS — Joint Commission Standards that Implicitly Address Ergonomics

➤ EP.1.10, Safety Management (EP1, EP4, EP6)
➤ HR.2.10, Initial Job Training; HR.2.20, Roles & Responsibilities; HR.2.30, Ongoing Education

To help organizations address the issues surrounding ergonomics, OSHA has taken a four-pronged approach. It has issued industry-specific ergonomic guidelines, developed an enforcement strategy, provided an outreach and assistance program, and encouraged additional research. Outreach and assistance is provided by OSHA to employers to promote awareness of the issues surrounding ergonomics and potential solutions. OSHA can assist and train employers, providing training grants targeted to ergonomics, and develop and provide distance learning courses. Because of a concern for immigrant worker safety, the guidelines are provided in Spanish, and potentially in other languages as well. OSHA intends to encourage researchers to develop methods to measure physical stress. OSHA has also established a national advisory committee on ergonomics to identify gaps between workplace needs and current research.

The first set of ergonomics guidelines developed by OSHA is for nursing homes. Issued on March 13, 2003, the guidelines specifically target the nursing home industry; however, they may be applicable to other industries, such as hospitals, assisted living facilities, and home care services. The guidelines contain a great deal of practical information that can be applied to other types of health care organizations, and therefore organizations may want to include them as part of a risk assessment process.

The stated goal of the nursing home guidelines is to reduce the number and severity of work-related MSDs. Accordingly, the guidelines make two primary recommendations:
- "Manual lifting of residents be minimized in all cases and eliminated when feasible."
- "Employers implement a systematic process for identifying and resolving ergonomics issues, and incorporate this process into its overall program to recognize and prevent work-related injuries and illnesses."

Developing a Process for Protecting Workers

When embarking on an ergonomics program, management of a health care organization should assign and communicate the responsibilities for establishing and managing the program. The designated individual or team should be given the authority, resources, and information necessary to fulfill the assigned responsibilities. Management should periodically communicate with organization employees about the ergonomics program and try to address employee concerns about MSDs. Finally, management should ensure that policies and practices do not discourage reporting of MSDs.

Employees should be active participants in the evaluation of the work area. They are the ones who know best how to do their jobs and they therefore have valuable input to provide. Employees should be encouraged to submit suggestions and concerns about the workplace; discuss the workplace and work methods; participate in the design of work, equipment, procedures, and training; evaluate equipment; and participate in surveys, task groups, and the program development process.[9]

If an employee develops a work-related MSD, prompt and effective management should be provided by the employer. This could include providing access to a qualified health care provider, who will provide a formal, written opinion of the case. Work restrictions or reassignment may be made as a result of the injury. In all cases, the injured employee should be afforded appropriate privacy of health-related information.

Chapter 3: Human Factor-Related Risks

To assist the health care provider with the assessment of the case, the organization should provide him or her with a description of the job activities of the affected employee to determine cause and effect. In addition, the provider could be provided with a listing of available alternative duty jobs in the event that the injured employee cannot return to his or her normal responsibilities due to the MSD.

Identifying Problems and Implementing Solutions

In an ergonomics program, identification of problems, or job hazard analysis, is a critical component. It involves evaluating the job in question to identify potential causative agents of MSDs. To do this, the performance of an employee who regularly performs the job should be observed. This observation should be followed with discussions or interviews with this employee and others to answer questions and hear their suggestions. The information obtained from this process should be analyzed to determine potential control measures that may be used to reduce the MSD risk.

As with other programs, OSHA and the Joint Commission would expect implementation of appropriate controls to address any identified hazards. Typically, these would include a combination of engineering, administrative, and work practice controls. Controls should be put in place and remain in force until the hazards are eliminated, reduced to an acceptable level or risk, or reduced to the extent feasible. It is also important that the organization periodically check for newly available controls that might further reduce the level of risk.

As previously mentioned, lifting and repositioning residents is a primary cause for MSDs. A primary focus of the following section relates to an assessment of the needs and abilities of the resident involved to determine the safest way to accomplish lifting and positioning.

When assessing a patient for lifting and positioning needs, organizations should consider the patient's required level of assistance, his or her size and weight, the ability and willingness of the resident to cooperate in lifting and repositioning, and other medical considerations.

To provide assistance with the assessment process, OSHA offers six flow charts (available at http://www.osha.gov) for varying types of transfers and repositions. These charts can help determine the best technique or type of device to assist with the resident movement. Tips are included regarding

Sidebar 3-3. Minimizing Patient Lifts

One organization has achieved a significant level of success with a program of "minimal lifts." Since 1998, the employees of Provena Health have sustained nearly 1,367 lower back injuries while moving patients or residents. Management of Provena Health (a Catholic health system that includes 6 hospitals, 16 long term care and senior residential facilities, 28 clinics, 5 home health agencies, and other health-related activities operating in Illinois and Indiana) estimates the cost of these employee back injuries to be $3.5 million.

In an effort to reduce injuries, Provena Health is instituting a new minimal lift environmental program in its hospitals and nursing homes. Instead of using manual transfers in which employees lift patients or residents, the organization will begin using mechanical equipment. "The program fits quite nicely with our service excellence initiative," said Paul Smith, system manager of the Workers' Compensation program.

As a result of the program, the network hopes to see greater safety for employees and patients, higher retention of clinical employees, and improved recruitment of clinical employees. Although funding for the $2.4 million program will come from a workers' compensation trust fund, Provena Health expects that these benefits will enable the program to pay for itself.[11]

helpful devices, the need for additional assistance, and cues that can be given to the resident to help the process along.

An important feature of the OSHA's ergonomics guidelines for nursing homes is an extensive section describing in detail various engineering controls to assist in transfers and repositions. Twenty-two different devices are illustrated and listed by the type of transfer, lift, or reposition for which each device is best suited. OSHA also offers a list of questions regarding the specifications of each device designed to assist health care organizations in selecting the appropriate device for the particular situation. The size and storage requirements of the assistive device are absolutely critical. OSHA notes, "If resident lifting equipment is not accessible when it is needed, it is likely that other aspects of the ergonomics process will be ineffective."

Although patient lifting and repositioning are significant issues to consider when designing an ergonomics program, other activities to consider include the following:
- Bending to make a bed or feed a resident
- Lifting above shoulder or below knee level
- Collecting waste
- Pushing heavy carts

PROTECTING THOSE WHO SERVE: Health Care Worker Safety

- Bending to remove linen from a deep cart
- Lifting and carrying
- Bending to manually crank an adjustable bed
- Removing laundry from washers and dryers

All of the above would be subject to a risk assessment process to determine if they are problematic for the particular organization. As with the lifting and positioning devices, OSHA does provide specific descriptions of controls available to address problems associated with these activities.

Training

After an ergonomics program is established, training is essential to make the program effective. Employers should provide information to employees about MSDs so that employees can recognize the signs and symptoms of them. Training should be presented in a language that employees can understand.

Although general ergonomics issues can be addressed in organizationwide training, the hazards found in each employee's job should also be addressed, making a department-specific training component important as well. For example, nursing assistants and others at risk of injury should be trained before they participate in any resident lifting or repositioning, or other activities that may put them at risk for MSDs. Demonstrations are particularly effective.

In addition to policies and procedures, it is important that employees understand early indications of MSDs so that they can be addressed promptly to avoid more serious injuries. Appropriate use of equipment and controls should also be covered, along with injury and illness reporting procedures.

Charge nurses and supervisors have the responsibility of enforcing safety and health programs, including ergonomics, with their staff. These nurses and supervisors are also likely to be the receivers of reports of injuries. They should be taught administrative details such as how to ensure that proper work practices are followed, and how to respond to reports of injuries. In addition, for identified problems in their work area, these staff members should understand how to help workers implement solutions.

Individuals who have been appointed as managers of ergonomics programs should be trained how to identify potential concerns and select solutions. Their responsibilities may include workplace and/or job observation and evaluation using various assessment tools. These people may participate in the selection of various pieces of equipment to address problems and assist in implementing this equipment. Finally, program evaluation is another training component of value for managers.[9]

Organizations must take ergonomics seriously. According to Dr. Fragala, "Organizations need to make the solutions to these problems a priority because of the impact of back injuries on the nursing force. Senior administrators need to examine closely the money and person-power that back injuries are costing them. When they do, they'll see that this is something on which they need to take immediate action to protect the people who are working in this profession."[7] The case study on this page discusses one organization's approach to ergonomics.

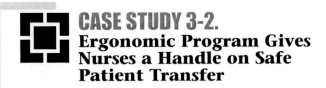

CASE STUDY 3-2.
Ergonomic Program Gives Nurses a Handle on Safe Patient Transfer

Veterans Health Administration Holds Up Back Pain

Meat packers. Coal miners. Garbage collectors. All have come and gone on the Bureau of Labor Statistics' list of top 10 at-risk occupations for musculoskeletal injuries. The only occupation seemingly permanently lodged on that list is nursing. More than half of all U.S. nurses suffer from chronic back pain, requiring 38% to take time off work and, perhaps most tellingly, causing 12% of them to leave the profession for good.

The crux of the problem is what it has always been: patients—moving them, lifting them, repositioning them.

Ten years ago, Audrey Nelson, Ph.D., R.N., F.A.A.N., director of the Veterans Health Administration (VHA) Patient Safety Research Center led a team of VHA researchers into battle against job-related musculoskeletal injuries in nursing. Based on the premise that there is no safe way to lift a dependent patient without assistive equipment, the comprehensive ergonomics program they developed has been proving itself in nursing homes for four years now and is beginning to penetrate the acute care hospital.

Technology, said Nelson, is the key to making it all work, but the other program elements add considerably to the chances of success. The program has eight elements:

- Ergonomic workplace assessments of patient care areas

- Patient assessment criteria (see Figure 3.9)
- Algorithms for safe patient handling and moving (see Figure 3.10)
- Equipment selection, storage, and maintenance
- Peer-safety leaders (Back Injury Resource Nurses or BIRN)
- Lifting teams
- After action reviews
- No-[manual]-lift policy

"We realized right away that we had to work with vendors to make the lifting equipment out there less cumbersome and easier to use, which has been done. In the last five or six years there's just been an explosion in technology to make patient handling safer," notes Nelson.

Investing in Infrastructure

Long term care (LTC) jumped on the program first, spurred by the release in 2003 of OSHA's "Guidelines for Nursing Homes—Ergonomics for the Prevention of Musculoskeletal Disorders," which were themselves based on the work of Nelson et al. The guidelines recommended that "manual lifting of patients be minimized in all cases and eliminated when feasible."

When the Orlando, Florida, VHA Healthcare Center opened its Nursing Home Care Unit in 1999, they did so with a "lift-free" policy in place, said Karen Putney, M.S.N., R.N., associate chief of nursing services. "But staff would always find a way to circumvent it because they felt it was faster for two of them to do the job manually."

Then Putney attended the first annual Safe Patient Handling and Movement Conference (http://www.cme.hsc.usf.edu) and heard Nelson explain that such policies don't work unless the infrastructure to support it is in place first—including adequate numbers and types of equipment for each high-risk unit, fully trained staff, and a supportive administration.

"So we installed 26 motorized over-the-bed lifts in about 28 rooms, which we reserve for our most dependent patients. We trained a BIRN for each unit who is responsible for training the other caregivers on the unit and designated a sort of super-BIRN who oversees the others and reviews all injuries. We made mechanized lifting skills part of our orientation and performance expectations for both nurses and aides."

They used a lot of strategies to "sell" the program, including posters, inservices, continuous reminders, and peer encouragement. But the key to gaining staff buy-in, she firmly believes, was to give staff hands-on input into the purchase of the equipment via an equipment fair.

"We asked staff to look over the equipment, try it out, evaluate it on a form, and then vote for the ones they liked best. Once the decision was made, we brought in the selected vendor to inservice staff."

Today, Putney said, the no-lift policy is given more than lip service. And they haven't had a back injury in a long time.

Adapting to the Acute Care Environment

The Orlando Nursing Home Care Unit was not alone in its success. The Patient Safety Center implemented the program on 25 high-risk units in Florida and Puerto Rico with "very positive" results, according to Nelson. In nine case studies evaluating the impact of lifting equipment in health care facilities, the incidence of injuries and the cost of workers' compensation both dropped by up to 95%.

With this kind of track record, it did not take long for the program to attract the interest of acute care hospitals. "The basic framework of the program can be the same in acute care," said Guy Fragala, Ph.D., P.E., C.S.P., director of compliance programs at Environmental Health and Engineering and a pioneering authority in the field of health care ergonomics. "But hospitals might need to make some adjustments to accommodate the needs of different environments, such as critical care and operating rooms. Overall you encounter more lateral transfers—bed-to-stretcher rather than bed-to-chair."

Also, where a resident in LTC might need to be reassessed periodically, the condition of a patient in a hospital can change rapidly. "Someone coming back from surgery can be totally dependent because of the anesthesia but only moderately dependent a couple of hours later – perhaps needing some help getting up – and a few hours after that, totally independent. So you need to do quicker, more frequent assessments in acute care."

PROTECTING THOSE WHO SERVE: Health Care Worker Safety

■■■ Figure 3-9. The Veterans Health Administration Patient Assessment Criteria

This form, which can easily be adapted for different settings, is available online as part of the VHA's ergonomics program at http://www.patientsafetycenter.com/Safe%20Pt%20Handling%20Div.htm.

**Assessment Criteria and Care Plan for
Safe Patient Handling and Movement**

I. **Patient's Level of Assistance:**
    _____ Independent — Patient performs task safely, with or without assistive devices.
    _____ Partial Assist — Patient requires no more help than stand-by, cueing, or coaxing, or no more than 50% physical assistance by the nurse.
    _____ Dependent — Patient requires more than 50% assistance by nurse, or is unpredictable in the amount of assistance offered.

An assessment should be made prior to each task if the patient has varying level of ability to assist due to medical reasons, fatigue, medications, etc. When in doubt, assume the patient cannot assist with the transfer/repositioning.

II. **Weight-Bearing Capability**
    _____ Full
    _____ Partial
    _____ No

III. **Upper Extremity Strength**
    _____ Yes
    _____ No

IV. **Patient's level of cooperation and comprehension:**
    _____ Cooperative — may need prompting; able to follow simple commands.
    _____ Unpredictable or varies (patient whose behavior changes frequently should be considered as "unpredictable", not cooperative, or unable to follow simple commands).

V. **Weight:** _____ **Height:** _____
Body Mass Index (BMI) [needed if patient's weight is more than 300]?: _____
If BMI exceeds 50, institute Bariatric Algorithms

The presence of the following conditions is likely to affect the transfer/repositioning process and should be considered when identifying equipment and technique needed to move the patient.

VI. **Check applicable conditions likely to affect transfer/repositioning techniques.**
    _____ Hip/Knee Replacements   _____ Postural Hypotension   _____ Amputation
    _____ History of Falls   _____ Severe Osteoporosis   _____ Urinary/Fecal Stoma
    _____ Paralysis/Paresis   _____ Splints/Traction   _____ Contractures/Spasms
    _____ Unstable Spine   _____ Fractures   _____ Tubes (IV, Chest, etc.)
    _____ Severe Edema   _____ Respiratory Compromise   _____ Severe Pain, Discomfort
    _____ Wounds Affecting Transfer/Positioning

Comments: _____

VII. Care Plan:

Algorithm	Task	Equipment/ Assistive Device	# Staff
1	Transfer To and From: Bed to Chair, Chair To Toilet, Chair to Chair, or Car to Chair.		
2	Lateral Transfer To and From: Bed to Stretcher, Trolley.		
3	Transfer To and From: Chair to Stretcher, or Chair to Exam Table.		
4	Reposition in Bed: Side-to-Side, Up in Bed.		
5	Reposition in Chair: Wheelchair and Dependency Chair.		
Bariatric 1	Bariatric Transfer To and From: Bed to Chair, Chair to Toilet, or Chair to Chair		
Bariatric 2	Bariatric Lateral Transfer To and From: Bed to Stretcher or Trolley		
Bariatric 3	Bariatric Reposition in Bed: Side-to-Side, Up in Bed		
Bariatric 4	Bariatric Reposition in Chair: Wheelchair, Chair or Dependency Chair		
Bariatric 5	Patient Handling Tasks Requiring Sustained Holding of a Limb/Access		
Bariatric 6	Bariatric Transporting (Stretcher, Wheelchair, Walker)		

Sling Type (circle choice):   Standard_____   Amputation_____   Head Support_____
Sling Size: _____

Signature: _____   **Date:** _____

[1] If patient's weight is more than 300 pounds, the BMI is needed. For online calculators, see: http://www.kcil.com/body_mass_index_calculator.html or http://www.sizewiserentals.com/bmicalculator.htm

These criteria are part of the Veterans Health Administration's comprehensive ergonomics program.

Source: Veterans Health Administration.

CHAPTER 3: HUMAN FACTOR-RELATED RISKS

■ ■ ■ Figure 3-10. The Veterans Health Administration's Patient Transfer Algorithm

This is one of a number of different algorithms available for use in implementing the VHA's ergonomics programs. See http://www.patientsafetycenter.com/Safe%20Pt%20Handling%20Div.htm.

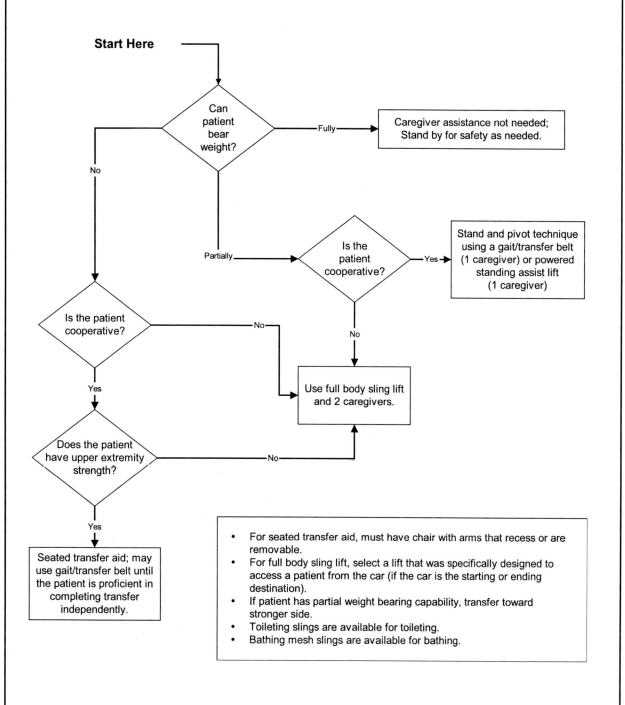

This algorithm is part of the Veterans Health Administration's comprehensive ergonomics program.

Source: Veterans Health Administration.

Winning over the Hospital Nurse

This is why nurses at Duke University Hospital in Durham, North Carolina, are asked to reassess patients at the start of every 12-hour shift when they take vitals, said Tamara James, M.A., C.P.E., director of ergonomics in Duke's Office of Occupational and Environmental Safety. They use decision guides provided by the vendor to help determine which piece of equipment is appropriate for each patient based on his or her current status.

Duke purchased 20 dependent lifts and 20 stand-assist devices, one of each for all of its adult inpatient units, and is about halfway through its roll-out of the program, which is a joint effort between nursing and ergonomics.

Initially the staff was skeptical, according to James. "They viewed it as just another thing they had to do and an additional piece of equipment they had to learn how to use. But I think now they are seeing the benefits. We've had some testimonials from nurses who say, 'You know, I get home at the end of the day and I don't feel like I've been beaten up,' and 'Now I feel like I can actually get through the rest of my career.'"

A bigger challenge, James said, was helping hospital administration appreciate the need for the program in the first place. "Our workers' comp costs were not especially high and there are so many competing priorities."

To bring the ergonomic issue up on the radar screen, program champions decided to look at patient satisfaction on the pilot unit. In the course of that study, they found that staff loved the lifts as much as the patients. "They were more comfortable and injuries were lower. Once administration understood this, it was very easy for them to say yes."

In fact, the hospital is now exploring the use of lifts in radiology, the ED, and some of its clinics.

High-end Technology, Quick ROI

In addition to ergonomic solutions that involve distinct pieces of equipment, such as patient lifts, Fragala pointed out that solutions can be built into the equipment hospitals are currently using, such as beds and chairs.

So if you spend $40,000 in equipment, there is a tremendous cost savings. Even on units where we've implemented these ceiling-mounted lifts on every single floor, the return on investment is less than two years. And the impact on recruitment and retention is phenomenal."[12]

EMERGENCY ACTION PLANNING

The Joint Commission defines an emergency as "a natural or manmade event that significantly disrupts the environment of care (for example, damage to the organization's building[s] and grounds due to severe winds, storms, or earthquakes); that significantly disrupts care, treatment, and services (for example, loss of utilities such as power, water, or telephones due to floods, civil disturbances, accidents, or emergencies within the organization or in its community); or that results in sudden, significantly changed or increased demands for the organization's services (for example, bioterrorist attack, building collapse, plane crash in the organization's community)."

Emergency management plans are extensively addressed in Joint Commission's accreditation standard, EC.4.10, with emergency drills separately addressed in EC.4.20. The actual requirement for the emergency management plan is in EP3: "The organization develops and maintains a written emergency management plan describing the process for disaster readiness and emergency management, and implements it when appropriate." EP4 goes on to add that the organization's leadership, including medical staff leadership in a hospital setting, must be involved with the development of the plan.

EC.4.10 includes 19 other elements of performance, all of which include various details of emergency planning that must be addressed by the health care organization to have a compliant plan. Organizations should review these elements of performance when creating an emergency plan to make sure all areas of emergency management and planning are addressed.

STANDARDS *Joint Commission Standards That Address Emergency Action Planning*

➤ EC.1.10, Safety Management; EC.4.10, Emergency Management (all EPs); EC.4.20, Emergency Drills
➤ HR.2.10, Initial Job Training (EP2); HR.2.20, Roles & Responsibilities; (EP3), HR.2.30, Ongoing Education (EP4)

Chapter 3: Human Factor-Related Risks

OSHA addresses emergency action planning in several standards and related documents.[†] Although the Joint Commission standards are obviously specific to health care, the OSHA standards are written for general industry. The overlap in the two agencies' requirements is significant, but the OSHA material does not contain all the depth necessary for managing an emergency event in a health care organization.

OSHA requires that an emergency action plan be written for all workplaces with ten or more employees; those with fewer employees may communicate the plan orally. Likewise, a written emergency management plan is required by Joint Commission for hospitals, ambulatory care, behavioral health care, and LTC organizations and laboratories.

Elements of an Emergency Action Plan

Both OSHA and the Joint Commission require organizations to assess what emergencies might reasonably occur in the workplace. As part of this assessment, organizations should consider how the need for the organization's services and the ability to provide those services will be impacted as well as the impact to the organization's employees.

After an assessment has been conducted, organizations should write an emergency management plan. Some elements of an emergency action plan include the following:

- Procedures for reporting an emergency
- Procedures for notifying employees of an emergency. The emergency management plan should address notification of employees, both on and off duty as per EC.4.10 EP7: "The plan provides processes for notifying staff when emergency response measures are initiated."

TIP ▶ Most often, on-duty staff are notified via a coded overhead page to specify the type of emergency. Off-duty staff, as needed, are usually called in based on a departmental roster. There are other ways to do this, such as notification via one or more specific radio station(s), a service that will call each employee and play a recorded message, or even a Web site posting.

[†] The titles of the standards are as follows:
  29CFR 1910.34 Coverage and Definitions
  29CFR 1910.38 Emergency Action Plans
All of these provide general, high level information about emergency planning, and 1910.34 states that every employee in general industry is covered, with the exception of mobile workplaces.[13]

Procedures for emergency evacuation, including type of evacuation and exit route assignments. In EC.4.10 EP12, the Joint Commission requires a process to evacuate a health care facility both horizontally and vertically, if necessary. If specific exit route assignments are necessary, they should be included in the organization's evacuation plan. (Note that area-specific fire evacuation routes are addressed in the fire response plan under EC.5.10 EP4.)

TIP ▶ Although OSHA suggests that workplace maps showing evacuation routes may be helpful, Joint Commission does not require the posting of evacuation routes. Employees in a health care organization should be responsible for directing patients and visitors in an emergency, and they are expected to be familiar with the routes. If maps are posted, however, they are expected to be current.

In addition to exit routes, safe areas of refuge for evacuation, such as a building divided by fire walls, should be considered.[14]

In health care facilities a complete evacuation is an extremely rare event that is seen as a last resort to manage an emergency. Due to the compartmentalization of health care facilities, these buildings are considered "defend in place" occupancies. Critical utility systems have backup sources (EC.4.10 EP20), and the buildings are not evacuated except in the most extreme situation. However, if an evacuation were to occur, organizations should have plans in place to identify who would stay behind to manage critical functions. Typically facilities management personnel would be designated via the departmental emergency plan to perform these functions:

- Description of the emergency command structure. Both the Joint Commission and OSHA require health care organizations during an emergency to function under a command structure that links with the community's command structure.
- Procedures to account for all employees after evacuation. In a health care organization, one must consider accounting for all patients as well as employees in an evacuation scenario. The issue of accounting for employees in an evacuation should be part of departmental plans.
- Sources of information about the plan or an explanation of employee duties under the plan. If employees have questions about the emergency plans in a health care organization, they typically ask their supervisor or department head. The

management plan may list an individual who is responsible for the plan, but that is not a Joint Commission requirement.

Training

Both the Joint Commission and OSHA expect role-specific training of all employees regarding their roles under the emergency management plan. Some training topics that may be helpful in this effort include the following:
- Individual roles and responsibilities
- Threats, hazards, and protective actions
- Notification, warning, and communications procedures
- Means for locating family members in an emergency
- Emergency response procedures
- Evacuation, shelter, and accountability procedures
- Location and use of common emergency equipment
- Location and use of PPE for specific emergency hazards
- Emergency shutdown procedures[15]

Plan Review

The Joint Commission has some requirements for review of the emergency management plan. EC.9.10 EP4 and EP5 call for an annual evaluation of the emergency management plan in terms of its objectives, scope, performance, and effectiveness. Based on this evaluation, and other assessments, such as critiques of all drills or newly received information, changes are made to the plan to keep it current. Supporting policies and procedures to the emergency management plan should receive at least a triennial review as per standard EC.1.10 EP6.

One way to look at the integration of all the components of an emergency action (or emergency management) plan is to see how it works in action. What follows is a case study showing a hospital response to a gas leak emergency.

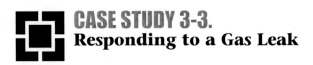

CASE STUDY 3-3. Responding to a Gas Leak

It is not surprising that at George Washington University Hospital (GW), the level-1 trauma center closest to the White House, emergency preparedness is an exceptionally high priority.

That preparedness paid off on the morning of October 7, 2003, when a gas leak occurred across the street from the hospital.

GW's response began when emergency management services (EMS) personnel on the ambulance ramp smelled gas, notified the hospital that the facility was being closed to ambulance traffic, and alerted both the fire department and the gas company. Shortly thereafter, a passing car burst into flames, and the street began to burn. When the fire department arrived, they entered the facility, ordered an evacuation via the public-address system, and began a floor-by-floor sweep.

"Fire departments need to be aware of the consequences of asking for a hospital evacuation," said John Rhodes, GW's trauma coordinator and chair of its multidisciplinary emergency management (EM) committee. That morning, they had approximately 400 patients—including both inpatient and outpatient—plus family members and hundreds of staff members.

The side of the hospital closest to the fire, including the emergency room, was cleared, with some ED patients transferred to other area hospitals. Approximately 120 people were moved to a nearby GW building, while other patients and family members were relocated to areas of the hospital farthest from the fire. Meanwhile, in the surgical unit, the chief medical officer took charge of decision making. Those surgeries that had not yet started were cancelled; those patients who had already been given anesthesia were held in the recovery area until they woke up. The surgeries in progress continued, with D.C. fire personnel nearby, monitoring for gas levels. If they'd detected a problem, the chief medical officer would have had to reconsider the course of the in-process surgeries.

"When emergency preparedness committees write their evacuation plans, they often don't think about who will make those kinds of medical decisions," Rhodes said, glad that GW had thought to include such a procedure in its plan. "It has to be someone with administrative powers as well as medical expertise."

In the case of GW's gas fire, the right people came together: The gas leak was sealed after about 40 minutes. Firefighters and hazmat crews put out the fire minutes later. And at approximately 12:00 p.m., the fire department gave the hospital the all-clear to move patients back into their rooms.

According to *The Washington Post*, some patients and staff reported the evacuation as a chaotic scene. And Rhodes somewhat agreed about the first few minutes of the response, attributing the panic to the evacuation order made via the public address system. "GW has an emergency paging system that can alert up to 85 key people at once—all the administrators, supervisors, and key resident physicians—without creating anxiety in everyone in the facility." Within minutes, this system was activated, allowing for more organization.

So what was the number one lesson learned during the gas fire emergency? Rhodes said, "All outside responding agencies need to know that (1) hospitals have their own emergency plans and (2) there is a designated person whom they should talk to: the person who will be making the decisions for the hospital." After this crucial communication connection is made, inside and outside responders can act as a team, making decisions jointly.

Rhodes acknowledged that EM planners face multiple challenges: First, it is expensive to have a good EM program. "It takes so many hours to do plans—hours of thinking, writing, meeting with equipment vendors." And emergency equipment is expensive—especially considering that it isn't used very often; with luck, maybe never. "But if you don't plan," Rhodes said, "it could be even more costly. Trying to make up plans as you move through an emergency is not ideal."

Second, without one or two vigorous EM champions in the organization, planning suffers. GW started disaster planning in the mid-1990s—in part due to the urging of two staff physicians with extensive EM experience responding to disaster situations both with FEMA and in hospitals all over the world. One of them was the original chair of D.C. Hospital Association's emergency management committee. Clearly, organizations benefit by cultivating an EM champion.

Rhodes also had other EM advice to share:
- EM plans must designate staff to liaison with outside agencies. During the gas fire, for example, one emergency medicine physician was assigned as liaison with EMS and coordinated transfers of patients to other facilities. Having these direct links between responders is key.

- EM plans must get everyone "talking the same language." During an emergency, outside responders don't necessarily know the name of the person who will be the EMS coordinator, but they need to know there will be one, so they can say, "Let me speak to the EMS coordinator." If Rhodes needs to contact the key person at the police or fire department, he needs to know who to ask for—not by name, but by title: the operations commander, for example. "That's what the Healthcare Emergency Incident Command System (HEICS) is for," Rhodes said. "So everyone uses the same terms."

Plans shouldn't delegate the entire responsibility for emergencies to the ED The whole hospital must be prepared—for example, with a plan for moving patients out of the ED as soon as possible so the ED is available to accept more victims.

Planners should include subacute hospitals and health care organizations in their planning process, because during an emergency, such facilities may become essential. For example, they may be able to accept less-acute patients from trauma centers, so that trauma center beds can be used for med-surge care. Until recently, many planners hadn't considered the importance of these other facilities.

Terrorism, said Rhodes, has helped the health care community prepare for all types of hazards. "It certainly helped us with the evacuation during the gas fire." [16]

The important lesson learned in the case study on pages 70-71 and in most other actual emergencies is that it is important for the emergency plans to be flexible so they can accommodate the nuances that occur with every scenario. They should be written at a high level to allow for decision making at the time of the event.

PERSONAL PROTECTIVE EQUIPMENT

PPE is the equipment that stands between the health care worker and the hazard when there is no other means to remove the hazard from the task or to reduce its intensity. PPE is the third level of control in OSHA's hierarchy of controls (discussed in Chapter One), following engineering, work practice, and administrative controls.

When one thinks of PPE in health care organizations, most likely protection against exposure to bloodborne pathogens comes to mind because that is one of the most frequently encountered hazards. But PPE is required to protect health care workers from more than just bloodborne pathogens. Large hospitals are like little cities, with individuals performing a variety of tasks, such as might be found across the spectrum of industries. Even small health care organizations still receive and store supplies, undergo construction and renovation, clean throughout their buildings, and may maintain a physical plant. All these areas may require workers to wear PPE.

PPE includes a variety of types of equipment such as eye and face protection, respiratory protection, head protection, extremity protection, and hearing protection. Although some of these types of protection are discussed in detail in other areas of this book, the following section provides an overview of PPE.

Standards and Requirements

The Joint Commission has several EC standards that address PPE. Its use is implicit in EC.1.10 EP1, which requires a safety management plan to "describe the processes it implements to effectively manage the environmental safety" of employees. EC.3.10 EP9 addresses hazardous materials spills and exposures and calls for procedures that include the specific protective equipment to be used. EC.1.10 EP4 states, "The organization conducts comprehensive, proactive risk assessments that evaluate the potential of adverse impact of buildings, grounds, equipment, occupants, and internal physical systems on the safety and health of patients, staff, and other people coming to the organization's facilities." Conducting a risk assessment to identify where PPE should be used would fall under this requirement.

STANDARDS — *Joint Commission Standards that Address Personal Protective Equipment*

▶ EC.1.10, Safety Management (EP1, EP4); EC.3.10, Hazardous Materials & Waste Management (EP9); EC.6.10, Medical Equipment Management; EC.7.10, Utilities Management
▶ HR.2.10, Initial Job Training; HR.2.20, Roles & Responsibilities; HR.2.30

OSHA has a series of standards addressing PPE.‡ The general requirements address the safe design of all equipment to be used, and the fact that the employer is responsible for ensuring that the PPE is adequate, appropriate, and properly maintained, even if it is owned by the employee. OSHA also requires that organizations conduct a hazard analysis regarding PPE to determine hazards present in an organization that could require PPE. OSHA also provides nonmandatory guidance to conduct the assessment.

When conducting a hazard assessment, consideration should be given to a variety of hazards and their sources, including:

- Impact: Sources of motion, such as machinery or processes where movement of tools or machinery could exist, or movement of personnel could result in impact with a stationary object
- Penetration: Sources of sharp objects that could cut or pierce body parts
- Compression: Sources of rolling or pinching objects. Sources of potential falling or dropping objects.
- Chemical: Sources of various chemical exposures
- Heat: Sources that would potentially result in burns, eye injury, or ignition of PPE
- Harmful dust sources
- Light (optical) radiation[17]

Organizations should analyze data obtained in a hazard assessment based on the type of hazard, level of risk, and seriousness of the potential injury. Based on familiarity with the hazards, the PPE available, and the environment in which it will be used, appropriate PPE should be selected. Again, this is a nonmandatory method of assessment. When the assessment is complete, the OSHA standard requires a written certification "that identifies the workplace evaluated, the person certifying that the evaluation has been performed, the date(s) of the hazard assessment, and that identifies the document as a certification of hazard assessment."[18]

Similarly to the workplace assessment to assign appropriate PPE, OSHA requires an assessment of the chemicals used in each laboratory procedure according to OSHA's Occupational Exposure to Hazardous Chemicals in Laboratories Standard, 29CFR 1910.1450

‡ OSHA's standards addressing PPE are as follows:
29CFR 1910.132	General requirements
29CFR 1910.133	Eye and face protection
29CFR 1910.134	Respiratory protection
29CFR 1910.135	Head protection
29CFR 1910.136	Occupational foot protection
29CFR 1910.137	Electrical protective devices

Figure 3-11. OSHA Standards That Require Employer-Provided PPE[19]

1910.28	Safety requirements for scaffolds
1910.66	Powered platforms for building maintenance
1910.94	Ventilation
1910.120	Hazardous waste operations and emergency response
1910.157	Portable fire extinguishers
1910.160	Fixed extinguishing systems, general
1910.242	Hand and portable powered tools and equipment, general
1910.243	Guarding of portable power tools
1910.252	General requirements (welding, cutting, and brazing)
1910.269	Electric power generation, transmission, and distribution
1910.1000	Air contaminants
1910.1003	13 carcinogens, and so on
1910.1096	Ionizing radiation
1910.95*	Occupational noise exposure
1910.134*	Respiratory protection
1910.146*	Permit-required confined spaces
1910.1001*	Asbestos
1910.1025*	Lead
1910.1030*	Bloodborne pathogens
1910.1047*	Ethylene oxide
1910.1048*	Formaldehyde

*Indicates PPE must be provided at no cost to the employee

This is only a partial listing of OSHA standards that may apply to health care.

Source: U.S. Department of Labor, Occupational Safety and Health Administration.

(e)(3)(ii). This assessment will lead to implementation of various controls as appropriate including PPE.

OSHA suggests that a workplace be reassessed periodically, to include a review of the occupational illness and injury records and a reassessment of the suitability of previously assigned PPE. All PPE should be inspected for condition and age.[19]

Other OSHA standards require PPE. A partial listing of which standards may apply to health care is provided in Figure 3-11.

Selection of PPE

When choosing the appropriate type of PPE, it is important to look at the hazards the PPE is trying to control. Figure 3-12 shows hazards that are particularly applicable to health care organizations and suggests possible PPE to address them.

Employers selecting PPE should take its fit and comfort into consideration and ensure that sizes are available to fit all necessary employees. It is important that PPE fits appropriately to be effective.

Some PPE is required by OSHA to meet American National Standards Institute (ANSI) standards. Such equipment includes eye and face protection, head protection, and foot protection.[19] To obtain copies of the ANSI standards, which are available for purchase, see their Web site at http://www.ansi.org.

There is no ANSI standard for hand protection, but a selection of appropriate gloves should be based on an evaluation of the task for which the gloves will be used and the material from which the gloves are made. Chemical exposures require an analysis of the chemical resistance of the glove material. Some types of glove materials and their characteristics are shown in Figure 3-13.§

---

§ An excellent table showing the resistance of Neoprene, Latex/Rubber, Butyl, and Nitrile gloves to specific chemicals is found in the OSHA 3151 publication.[19]

Figure 3-12. Hazard Category Descriptions

CATEGORY	POTENTIAL HAZARDS	POSSIBLE PPE
Impact	Injuries resulting from such things as slips, falls, objects falling on employees, things piled too high causing them to fall onto employees, things (such as carts and wheelchairs) running into employees, failure to use seat belts in motor vehicles, and so on.	Slip-resistant footwear Hard hats in construction areas Seat belts and so on
Penetration	Invasive injuries resulting from needlesticks, cuts from sharps, splashes to eyes, and so on.	Eye protection Gloves Face shields and so on
Compression	Injuries to feet, hands, and so on as a result of objects (such as carts and wheelchairs,) rolling over them.	Hand protection Foot protection
Chemical	Injuries from improper use of chemicals of any kind.	Eye protection Gloves Aprons Respiratory protection and so on
Heat	Injuries from fire, flammable gases, steam and/or other sources of extreme heat.	Eye protection Hand/arm protection and so on
Harmful Dust	Potential harm from inhaling dust and/or other harmful airborne particles, such as TB bacteria, asbestos, lead, or wood shavings.	Respiratory protection Eye protection and so on
Light	Injuries from improper use of lasers, welding equipment and/or other harmful light.	Eye protection and so on
Bloodborne Pathogens	Injuries/illnesses resulting from exposure to blood, body fluids, and/or other potentially infectious material.	Eye/face protection Shoe covers Gloves Gowns and so on
Noise	Injuries resulting from exposure to machinery or equipment emitting loud and/or damaging sounds.	Hearing protection and so on

These hazards are particularly applicable to health care and may be addressed by the PPE noted.
Source: U.S. Department of Labor, Occupational Safety and Health Administration.

Chapter 3: Human Factor-Related Risks

■ ■ ■ Figure 3-13. Glove Materials and Their Characteristics[19]

Butyl (synthetic rubber)	Protect against variety of chemicals Resist oxidation Flexible at low temperatures
Natural Latex Rubber	Comfortable Good tensile strength, elasticity, temperature resistance May cause allergic reactions; hypoallergenic alternatives available
Neoprene (synthetic rubber)	Pliable Good finger dexterity Tear resistant Chemical and wear resistance better than natural rubber
Nitrile	Protection from chlorinated solvents Good dexterity and sensitivity Stand up to heavy use

Not all gloves give equal protection.
Source: U.S. Department of Labor, Occupational Safety and Health Administration.

PPE Use

PPE should be donned before contact with a patient, and generally before entering the patient's room. When patient contact has been completed, it should be removed and discarded carefully, either at the doorway or immediately outside the patient's room. Hand washing should be performed immediately. If respiratory protection is being used (see the following section), it should only be removed after leaving the room.

If using multiple pieces of PPE, an individual should put on his or her gown first, then mask or respirator, goggles or face shield, and finally gloves. This sequence is subject to practical judgment with different combinations of PPE.

Training

After PPE selections are made, organizations should train employees on the equipment. Topics may include the following:
- When PPE is necessary
- What PPE is necessary
- How to properly don, doff, adjust, and wear PPE
- Limitations of the PPE
- Care, maintenance, useful life, and disposal of the PPE[18]

Training must be done before the employee performs any work requiring the PPE, and must be repeated if there is a demonstrated lack of understanding, if the job has changed, or if the PPE has changed. The Joint Commission will assess employee training by asking staff members to describe or demonstrate their knowledge of appropriate PPE. OSHA requires that "The employer shall verify that each affected employee has received and understood the required training through a written certification that contains the name of each employee trained, the date(s) of training, and that identifies the subject of the certification."[18]

To see how all the aspects of a PPE program work together under extreme circumstances, consider the case study on page 75, which looks at an infectious disease outbreak in a LTC setting.

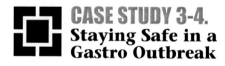

CASE STUDY 3-4.
Staying Safe in a Gastro Outbreak

A norovirus is a remarkably hardy and potent organism. It can remain infectious on environmental surfaces for days, and has one of the lowest infectious doses of any agent that causes gastroenteritis. Millions of particles are present in the stool and vomitus of someone who is ill, and the illness is characterized by frequent, often projectile vomiting.

All of this means that maintaining a clean environment during an outbreak of norovirus is critically important to managing an organization's safety risks, as required in EC.1.0. It is also—as many cruise ship lines can testify—a very difficult task, even when the affected population is ready and able to cooperate. Due to dementia, most of the patients at the 120-bed Nursing Home Care Unit (NHCU) #1, in the Livermore Division of the Palo Alto Healthcare System, Palo Alto, California, are neither.

Infection control practitioner Gina Oda, M.S., C.I.C., had little doubt that norovirus, typically a wintertime bug, was the culprit when nursing staff contacted her early in February 2003 about short-lived cases of vomiting with rapid recovery on Unit 1B. Among the first calls she made was to Thomas J. Fitzgerald III, C.H.E.S.P., chief of the system's environmental management service (EMS) and the current president of the American Society for Healthcare Environmental Services (ASHES).

A Sense of Ownership

Along with presentation and duration, the epidemic curve would turn out to be classic for norovirus as well (see Figure 3-14). Oda explains that, thanks to the home's "fantastic documentation," which features computerized chart notes on every patient almost every day, including any change in status, she was easily able to track the outbreak from its beginning on January 31 of that year.

"The first two cases were separated by a few days, so nobody thought anything about it. And then *boom*—all of a sudden we had a number of new cases, until the illness peaked around mid-February and then started gradually to go down. The last straggler case was on February 20." All told, 41 of 77 patients—almost all on the two units occupying the second of the home's two floors—and 30 of 109 staff were affected.

Without question, said Oda and Fitzgerald, these numbers would have been higher, the spread of the illness wider, had their two departments not had a solid history of teamwork. The fact that housekeeping staff had already been trained in basic infection control concepts and instilled with a sense of ownership in patient outcomes made it easier for the nursing home to implement early and effective control measures, as required by IC.1.10, EP1, in the case of all health care–associated infections (HAI).

These measures, of course, included PPE for all staff. In addition to goggles and gloves, which they wear all the time, housekeepers were asked to wear gowns and masks while on the units affected. Nurses donned face protection, goggles and/or masks, when interacting with patients who were actively ill.

The system had not yet completed installation of handrub dispensers in all patient and common rooms in its nursing homes. So Oda made sure that all staff, including housekeeping staff, were supplied with pocket-sized containers of handrub for personal use in keeping their hands clean.

Dementia Complicates Control Issues

As recommended by California's Department of Health Services Division of Communicable Disease Control, control measures also included the following:

- Minimize movement of patients
- Cancel or postpone all group activities
- Limit movement of staff between units to the extent possible
- Ask staff who become infected to stay home for four days
- Ask visitors not to visit if they or the person they are visiting is sick, and to wear gloves and wash their hands thoroughly when on the unit. (Because social needs are paramount in the care of persons with dementia, isolation from outsiders is not always possible.)
- Reassign unit volunteers unless they are performing essential tasks
- Close the unit to new admissions and discharge any patients well enough to go home

What might seem reasonable on a general medical or surgical ward can be highly problematic in a nursing home. For example, while it would clearly be desirable to restrict patients to their rooms, most activities in a LTC setting are done in groups, including eating meals. Staff did serve all meals to patients in their individual rooms during the outbreak. They deliberately used disposable trays, dishes, and utensils, which were bagged up for disposal in infectious waste cans placed in individual rooms and around the units, thus sparing kitchen staff from exposure to the virus.

Chapter 3: Human Factor-Related Risks

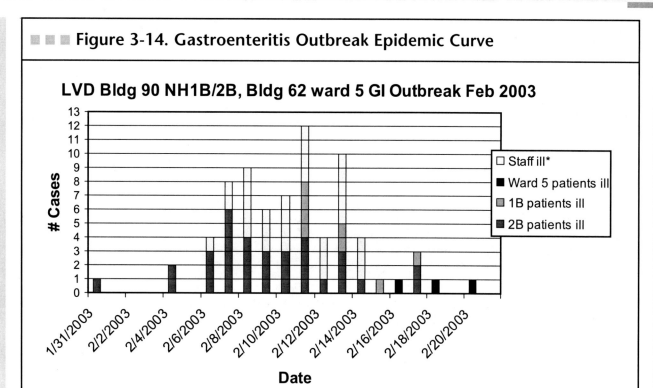

Figure 3-14. Gastroenteritis Outbreak Epidemic Curve

In classic norovirus fashion, the outbreak, which ran from January 31 to February 20, started slowly, then accelerated dramatically.

Source: Nursing Home Care unit #1, Livermore division, Palo Alto Healthcare System, CA.

But the fact is, as Fitzgerald explained, patients with dementia "are on the go all the time, walking up and down the halls, touching things, touching each other. You can't isolate them completely and you can't explain to them what's happening. You can't get them to understand the need to avoid touching their mouths or their friends."

For this reason, he considers the recreation therapy staff to be among the heroes of the outbreak. They did not go into rooms where patients were actively ill and they protected themselves by wearing gowns and gloves. But "by working with the other patients individually to make sure they had magazines, puzzles, and human contact on a regular basis, they were able to keep people in their rooms to a great extent and still keep things under control."

But it was the housekeeping staff, working hand-in-glove with nursing and administration, who kept the norovirus itself under

Case at a Glance

Main Challenge: To protect worker safety along with patients during an outbreak of norovirus in a nursing home.

Issues: Nursing Home Care Unit #1 in the Livermore Division of the VA Palo Alto Healthcare System is populated primarily by patients suffering from dementia, who pose special control challenges.

Joint Commission Standards:
EC.1.10. The health care organization manages safety risk.
EC.1.10 EP5. The health care organization uses the risks identified to select and implement procedures and controls to achieve the lowest potential for adverse impact on the safety and health of patients, staff, and other people coming to the hospital's facilities.
IC.1.10, EP1, An organizationwide IC program is implemented.

Solutions: The nursing home implemented a campaign of constant cleaning, upgraded personal protective measures, and reduced census.

Outcomes: The outbreak was fully contained in three weeks, with incidence among staff limited to 27.5%.

control, protecting health care professionals and the patients alike with their "goal-line stance on cleaning," as Fitzgerald described it.

Bucket Brigade

Normally two housekeepers are on each of the two units affected by the outbreak, working eight hours a day. As soon as Fitzgerald got the call from Oda about the outbreak, they started cleaning almost around the clock.

"We had people work overtime for three or four hours in the evening and we had people come in early, two to three hours before the shift started, when the patients started to get up." Using rags might have meant exposing laundry staff to the virus, so the housekeepers armed themselves with buckets of quat disinfectant and rolls of wet task wipes. They cleaned heavily in the bathrooms and living spaces and moved up and down the halls, wiping down surfaces in the unit's common contact areas continually. Hand railings, door knobs, and other objects frequently touched by hands were the focus of special attention.

Buckets of disinfectant were also placed in each patient room so that nursing staff could clean surfaces as necessary between regular cleanings.

Oda noted that, in line with several recent reports in the literature that norovirus can actually tolerate a certain amount of quat, the nursing home would probably use a chlorine solution in a similar situation in the future.

Keeping Communication Lines Open

As in so many crises in health care settings, interdisciplinary communication and cooperation were key to the home's success in squelching the outbreak. "It isn't just a matter of IC coming in and telling everybody what to do," Oda explained.

"We work very closely with the chief nurse of extended care, the physicians and other providers, along with the housekeeping staff. We've established good relationships that involve a lot of give and take. Our role is to assess the situation and prioritize what's needed in order to keep staff, as well as patients, safe. Sometimes we have to make recommendations that will be difficult for staff to carry out and they let us know what help they need."

Group meetings, in which Oda and Fitzgerald met with lead staff in nursing, social work, and recreation therapy, were held several times during the outbreak. Oda considers these essential to head off snafus that can come up when people rely exclusively on phone and e-mail. The nurse practitioner for the system's Livermore Division held inservices for all staff, reinforcing the requirements for control of norovirus.

At the same time, said Fitzgerald, EMS staff met with their own supervisors to discuss strategy and keep on top of the situation. "Supervisors passed along all the information they received from IC about how many patients were getting sick, how many days we had had without new cases, etc. They also gave them positive feedback on the job they were doing.

"I know they were very proud to help during this outbreak, and I was proud of them. I always let my housekeepers know that it takes every entity in the facility to keep HAI at bay. Their cleaning keeps the direct care staff safe, so the direct care staff can care for the patients."[20]

Decontamination

One aspect of PPE that many health care organizations, hospitals in particular, wrestle with is identifying which type of equipment is appropriate for performing decontamination activities. Joint Commission's standard EC.4.10 EP21 states that the emergency management plan "identifies means for radioactive, biological, and chemical isolation and decontamination." This EP is applicable only to hospitals, ambulatory care organizations, and LTC organizations.

The Joint Commission does not designate one particular way of performing decontamination activities. Although this requirement has been present in the standards for some time, many organizations have addressed it in the past by deferring to a fire department hazardous materials team or designating one hospital in the community to provide decontamination services. Since the terrorist attacks of September 11, 2001, however, the issue of decontamination has taken on a new emphasis.

A variety of approaches to PPE for decontamination have been suggested and much research has been done on this issue. Some organizations feel that

CHAPTER 3: HUMAN FACTOR-RELATED RISKS

Level A or B PPE is necessary for an unidentified exposure. However, these high levels of protection present significant disadvantages to employees wearing them, and may present hazards themselves.

In December 2004 OSHA published a new document, "OSHA Best Practices for Hospital-Based First Receivers of Victims from Mass Casualty Incidents Involving the Release of Hazardous Substances." As its title suggests, this document does not provide regulatory requirements, but rather guidance based on best practices currently in use in the field. Although the scope of this publication does not allow an in-depth discussion of the OSHA document, it is highly recommended that hospital personnel involved with emergency planning read the document in its entirety. In the document, OSHA discusses PPE selection and employee training for participation in decontamination activities. It contains a table of minimum recommended PPE for both the hospital decontamination zone and the post-decontamination zone, provided that certain prerequisite conditions are met.

RESPIRATORY PROTECTION

When thinking about respiratory protection in health care organizations, probably the first thing that comes to mind is the use of respirators to protect against exposure to tuberculosis (TB). These respirators represent the most common use, but should not be the only respirators covered under an organization's respiratory protection program. Other health care activities that may require the use of a respirator include decontamination processes, asbestos removal, ethylene oxide use, formaldehyde use, and exposure to other hazardous chemicals or drugs, to name a few.

A respirator is much more than a surgical mask. It is a piece of PPE, used when engineering controls cannot remove hazardous atmospheres in the work area. A respirator must cover at least the nose and the mouth, if not the entire face or head of the wearer, to protect against hazards in the atmosphere that could lead to various occupational diseases such as cancer, lung diseases, and so forth.

Standards and Regulations

The Joint Commission implicitly addresses respiratory protection in several of its standards. As with many of the topics discussed in this publication, respiratory protection for employees is presumed under EC.1.10, which calls for effective management of environmental safety for all individuals, including staff members. In the EC.3.10 standard on hazardous materials and waste management, there are several related elements of performance. EP2 calls for a hazardous materials inventory consistent with applicable law and regulation for those materials used, stored, or generated. That is followed by a requirement in EP3 for processes to cover, among other things, handling and using chemicals, and EP8 addresses the monitoring and disposing of hazardous gases and vapors.

STANDARDS *Joint Commission Standards that Implicitly Address Respiratory Protection*

➤ EC.1.10, Safety Management; EC.3.10, Hazardous Materials & Waste Management (EP2, EP3, EP8)
➤ R.2.20, Roles & Responsibilities (EP3); HR.2.30, Ongoing Education (EP4)

OSHA has one respiratory protection regulation, 29CFR 1910.134. Within this regulation, OSHA requires a full respiratory protection program in all workplaces where respirator use is required. The defined objective of this program is to prevent occupational illness due to exposure to air contaminated with harmful dusts, fogs, fumes, mists, gases, smokes, vapors, or sprays. The contents of such a program must include:
- Written worksite-specific procedures
- Program evaluation
- Selection of an appropriate respirator approved by the National Institute for Occupational Safety and Health (NIOSH)
- Training
- Fit testing
- Inspection, cleaning, maintenance, and storage
- Medical evaluation
- Work area surveillance
- Air quality standards[21]

The case study on page 80 discusses the particular aspects of one organization's respiratory protection program.

PROTECTING THOSE WHO SERVE: Health Care Worker Safety

CASE STUDY 3-5.
A Respiratory Protection Program for Worker Safety

During the summer of 2003, the world watched as the SARS virus hop scotched its way from China to Hong Kong to Canada. In the process, it infected nearly 8,500 people from 29 countries. The epidemic claimed 813 lives, a fatality rate of 9.6%. Of the total number of likely cases reported by the World Health Organization, 21% were health care workers.

These statistics prompted officials at the University of Maryland Medical Center in Baltimore to reexamine the role of the medical center's respiratory protection program in isolating infectious agents. Those agents might include SARS, tuberculosis, a bioterrorism threat, or an emerging pathogen such as avian influenza. "Although we had confidence in our existing respiratory protection program, we decided to review and strengthen it to meet the wide-ranging new threats to health care workers," said Craig D. Thorne, M.D., M.P.H., F.A.C.P., F.A.C.O.E.M., the medical director of employee health and safety at the medical center.

First Comes the Policy

The first step was to write a new policy outlining the parameters of a respiratory protection program that complies with OSHA 29 CFR 1910.134. This OSHA standard contains complete guidelines for any employer setting up a respiratory protection program.

Linda Pelletier, R.N., M.B.A., the medical center's emergency response planner, and her colleagues drafted a policy that includes everything OSHA requires, including selection and use of respirators, medical evaluation, fit testing, maintenance, disinfection, and distribution of respiratory protection. The policy applies not just to medical center employees but also to contract workers such as physicians, campus police, students, volunteers, and traveling nurses. "We made sure our policy was comprehensive and seamless so it would comply with OSHA and Joint Commission standards," said Thorne.

Pelletier is also the administrator of the organization's Respirator Program. She is responsible for making sure the policy is implemented, reviewed, and monitored. She's also responsible for training employees to use respiratory protection.

Thorne created a training sheet showing the two types of respirators used at the medical center and a separate sheet illustrating and explaining the components of each respirator so users can check their respirator before using it. "We use the training sheet to acquaint workers with the respirators," said Pelletier, "and then do hands-on skills training to make sure workers know how to use them."

A Phased Approach to Training

The medical center used a phased approach to train its health care workers. "Even before the policy was fully approved," Thorne recalled, "we started implementing it on an interim basis. That way, if there were an incident such as a SARS epidemic or a flu outbreak, we'd have enough workers trained and equipped to deal with it." The medical center designated a sample staff of physicians, nurses, university police, respiratory therapists, and radiology technicians who were all medically cleared, fit

---

Case at a Glance

Main Challenge: Design, implement, and monitor a comprehensive program of respiratory protection for all workers at the University of Maryland Medical Center in Baltimore to protect against airborne infectious diseases such as SARS, TB, influenza, or even bioterrorist threats.

Issues: Train nearly 5,000 workers—including staff and contractors, from physicians to housekeeping—to use respiratory protection.

Joint Commission Standards: EC.1.10 The health care organization manages safety risks. EC.1.10 EP 5 The health care organization uses the risks identified to select and implement procedures and controls to achieve the lowest potential for adverse impact on the safety and health of staff.

Solutions: Offer medical clearance, fit testing, and training to all workers.

Outcome: The medical center is now on track to train and equip all personnel to use respiratory protection in case of any outbreaks of infectious diseases.

tested, and trained to use respiratory protection. Then, over time, the medical center increased the number of qualified workers. The medical center pre-assigns respirators to certain high-risk areas, such as emergency medicine, ambulatory care, internal medicine, the ICUs, and the morgue.

Pelletier explained to many workers that a surgical mask offers no respiratory protection and that they must use one of two different kinds of respirators. The N-95 is a disposable respirator that protects against infectious droplets but not against chemicals or gases; it fits tightly to the face and requires fit testing. The other type is a powered air-purifying respirator (PAPR), which features a hood, filters, tubing, a cartridge, and a battery; although the PAPR requires a medical clearance, it doesn't require fit testing.

The fit testing of the N-95 takes about 30 minutes per worker, and Pelletier handled much of the testing herself. The medical center found that many of its nurses and other clinical workers are excellent teachers. So as part of a "train-the-trainer" program, Pelletier trained nurses and senior partners in several departments to do much of the fit testing of their employees. This tactic helped roll out the protection program quickly and efficiently. In addition, the medical center hired a medical technician to assist Pelletier with fit testing. The facility currently has 6,000 respirators in storage, including PAPRs and N-95s, for use on demand.

Because a medical clearance is required to use the PAPR, workers start by completing the mandated OSHA Respirator Medical Evaluation Questionnaire, which must then be reviewed by a licensed health care provider, such as a physician, a nurse/practitioner, or a physician assistant. In the start-up phase of the program, those questionnaires were assessed by volunteer physicians at the medical center under the direction of Employee Health Services. But because the medical center wanted all 5,000 workers covered by the respiratory protection program, it began looking for cost-effective options. The medical center decided to have the assessments handled by an online service at a cost of $25 each. Less than 1% of the online clearances required a follow-up physical by a clinician.

Because of concerns about bioterrorist agents, the medical center's respiratory protection program has been supplemented with grant money from the Health Resources and Services Administration (HRSA) of the Department of Health and Human Services (HHS). In addition, OSHA requires organizations to keep detailed records showing which employees have been medically cleared, fit tested, and trained.

A Hierarchy of Protection

Thorne sees respiratory protection as one element in a hierarchy of protection against airborne infection. "The highest level of this program," said Thorne, "is using engineering controls to separate the infectious agent from each individual. So we looked at our isolation capacity, and we made sure that we have negative pressure isolation rooms in the Emergency Department and other areas of the hospital."

The next level in the hierarchy is work practice controls to limit the number of health care workers entering an infectious patient's room. The third level is PPE. Thorne said, "We see respiratory protection as a vital supplement to the other two levels of protection for workers and patients."

Words to the Wise

Thorne and Pelletier offer several tips to organizations that may be considering instituting or upgrading their respiratory protection program. They recommend starting with the e-tools at the OSHA Web site at http://www.osha.gov because of the expense of taking doctors and nurses away from their patient-care duties. For her part, Pelletier advises working closely with Infection Control and Biomedical Equipment and Distribution to make sure that staff members follow the latest guidelines from the CDC for cleaning and disinfecting the respirators. And because PAPR respirators include multiple components, Pelletier recommends coordinating carefully with biomed equipment experts to make sure that the PAPR units arrive with all attachments intact and with the batteries charged, and are tested for air flow after they have been inspected visually. Each unit should also include an instruction pamphlet showing how to use it, along with a phone number where recipients can set up retraining and request additional units.

Thorne describes the medical center's senior management as very supportive of the respiratory program. "They realize the importance of our respiratory protection program in promoting the health and safety of everyone concerned," he said, "from workers to patients to visitors."[22]

Respirator Selection

Two different kinds of respirators are available. Tight fitting respirators fit to the facial contours of the wearer. They may be half masks, which cover the nose and mouth, or full face, which cover the entire face as implied. Loose fitting respirators completely cover the head with a hood or helmet.

Respirators may be divided into classes based on their operation. Air-purifying respirators remove contaminants from the air in the work location using filters, cartridges, or canisters. There are three types of air-purifying respirators:

- Particulate respirators capture dust, mist, and fume particles, but are not effective against gases or vapors. They become more effective as particles accumulate on the filter, but this will eventually lead to difficulty breathing. The filters should be replaced when that happens.
- Combination respirators are effective against both particulates and gases. They have both types of filters, but may be heavy to wear.
- Gas and vapor respirators are used against gas and vapors as the name implies. They must have filters (cartridges) specifically for removal of the contaminant in question and be color coded accordingly. When the cartridges' absorbing capacity is depleted, they are no longer effective and must be changed. This can be done on a predetermined schedule to prevent any employee exposure. Some cartridges have an "end of service life indicator" (ESLI) that provides an indication that they must be changed.[23]

Atmosphere-supplying respirators actually supply clean air to the wearer from a self-contained tank or via a connection to an air supply system of cylinders or air compressors. Employers are required to provide high-quality breathing gases. For purposes of decontamination, *NFPA 99, Health Care Facilities*, also permits the connection to piped medical air, providing an assessment has been made that doing so will not interfere with patient needs. Atmosphere-supplying respirators may be subdivided into the following groups:

- Air-supplying respirators use a hose from a fixed air supply source. They can be effective for long periods of time and are light weight, but limit mobility due to the tether.
- Combination respirators have an air supply as just described, but also a small auxiliary self-contained tank, providing only enough air to escape during an emergency. They are often used in confined space entry and may be used where the work atmosphere can be or is immediately dangerous to life or health.
- Self-contained breathing apparatus (SCBA) have a wearable air supply pack to provide air for 30 minutes to 4 hours, depending on the type. While they are heavy to wear, they do not restrict motion because they have no tether connection.[23]

Beyond the contaminant itself, other factors should be considered in respiratory selection. The size and activity in the work area will have an influence on the respirator used. Some areas may be too small to effectively maneuver using SCBA. In an area of high equipment use, an air-supplying respirator may not be practical due to the hose connection. Because respiratory protection may be difficult to wear, employee factors, such as medical conditions (see medical evaluation section) and comfort should also be considered. Each type of respirator has pros and cons. All respirators selected for use must be NIOSH-certified for the use to which they will be applied.

The OSHA Respiratory Protection e-Tool[23] has information on selecting the proper respirator for the exposure, and even has a section called "Advisor Genius" that will lead to the correct selection via a series of directed questions.

Medical Evaluation

Breathing through a respirator is not as easy as regular breathing. Negative pressure respirators (air pressure inside the face piece is negative relative to ambient air) restrict breathing, SCBA are heavy to wear, and some respirators may cause claustrophobia. Due to the challenges associated with respirator breathing, OSHA requires a medical evaluation of each employee to determine his or her ability to use a respirator, prior to being fit tested. Although this is not surveyed by the Joint Commission, the OSHA mandate must be followed by organizations using respiratory equipment.

According to OSHA, a medical evaluation must be performed by a physician or other licensed health care professional, but that does not necessarily imply a medical examination is required. The evaluation must be done using a mandatory medical questionnaire that is available in Appendix C of the OSHA respiratory protection standard.[24] Note the optional questions that may be added at the end of the questionnaire. When conducting the examination, the physician should have several pieces of information available including the type and weight of the respirator to be used, the duration and frequency of respirator use, the expected physical work effort, any additional protective clothing and equipment to be worn, the temperature and humidity extremes that may be encountered, and a copy of the written respiratory protection program.[25] The individual performing the medical evaluation is required to provide a written recommendation about the employee's ability to use a respirator and any limitations to its use.

According to OSHA, the questionnaire must be administered confidentially during normal working hours at a convenient time and place. The employee must have the opportunity to discuss the questionnaire and its results with the physician or other administrator, and request a follow up medical examination if a need is determined. This follow up exam may include testing, other diagnostics, and consultation as necessary.

The medical evaluation must be repeated if any applicable changes in the employee or in workplace conditions arise.

Fit Testing

Because tight fitting respirators must seal to the face of the wearer, a fit test of each employee should be done prior to his or her use of the respirator. Facial hair can interfere with the respirator seal, and many employers therefore have rules prohibiting facial hair if respirator use is required. Eyeglasses may also interfere with the seal, as may facial deformities, the absence of normally worn dentures, or jewelry.

The fit test may be either qualitative or quantitative. A qualitative fit test uses a harmless substance that either has an odor or is irritating. This substance is introduced into the breathing zone around the respirator being worn. If the person wearing the respirator can detect the substance, the respirator does not fit properly. A quantitative fit test is more accurate. It requires the wearer to perform exercises that could cause leakage around the face piece, and an instrument measures the amount of leakage into the respirator. Detailed mandatory fit testing procedures are included in Appendix A[26] of the OSHA respiratory protection standard. OSHA requires fit testing to be repeated annually.

Respiratory Protection for Tuberculosis

The issue of annual fit testing is controversial at the time of this writing with respect to respiratory protection for TB. Currently, respiratory protection for TB is addressed in the same OSHA standard as all other respiratory protection. This requires an annual fit test for all staff members who would need respiratory protection if exposed to an individual with suspected or confirmed TB. In most health care environments, this is a rare occurrence, but many staff members need to be fit tested for respirator use to account for a possible exposure. An annual fit test under these circumstances can be a costly proposition.

A number of professional organizations, including the Association for Professionals in Infection Control and Epidemiology (APIC) and the American Hospital Association, argued against the necessity of an annual fit test for TB to ensure safety for staff. Although the annual fit test requirement is in the OSHA standard, the current status is that in the fiscal year 2005 omnibus spending bill, there is a provision prohibiting OSHA from enforcing the annual fit testing requirement for occupational exposure to tuberculosis in health care facilities. This is in effect through September 30, 2005. It also contains advisory language for OSHA not to take additional action on this issue until the CDC completes the current revision of its TB guidelines.[27]

Seal Check

Each time an employee uses a respirator following the fit test, he or she must perform a "seal check" to ensure a good seal between the respirator and the face. Organizations can use OSHA suggestions regarding how to conduct an appropriate seal test; however, manufacturer-recommended seal check procedures are also acceptable to OSHA.

Training

All employees who are required to use respirators must be trained in their use and limitations. Employees should be taught that improper respirator use or maintenance can lead to exposure. According to OSHA requirements, training must occur prior to the initial use of a respirator, unless training has been provided within the past year by another employer. Following are some areas to include in the training process:
- The reason(s) for respirator use
- The nature of the respiratory hazard and potential consequences of improper fit, use, or maintenance

- Limitations and capabilities of the respirator
- Use in emergency situations
- How to inspect the respirator, put it on, remove it, use it, and check the seals
- Procedures for maintenance and storage
- Recognition of medical signs and symptoms that may limit or prevent effective use

Retraining should be done annually and when there are changes in workplace conditions, new types of respirators used, or there is an indication that retraining is needed based on the employee's knowledge or performance.

Respirator Maintenance

Respirators must be inspected for wear and tear before and after each use. Particular attention should be paid to rubber or plastic parts that can deteriorate or lose pliability. The tightness of all connections should be checked.

If SCBAs are being used, they should be inspected at least monthly. Chemical cartridges and canisters should be replaced as indicated or specified to ensure they are providing complete protection. Mechanical filters should be replaced as necessary to prevent high resistance to breathing.

Disposable respirators must be assigned to only one individual. Reusable respirators must be cleaned and disinfected as often as necessary to keep them in sanitary condition. This would include before being worn by different individuals and immediately after each use for emergency-use respirators and those used for fit testing.

Respirators should be washed in a detergent solution and then immersed in a disinfectant solution. OSHA has specific requirements for cleaning and disinfecting respirators; alternately, manufacturer's cleaning procedures may be used.

Respirator storage should protect them from dust, sunlight, heat, extreme cold, excessive moisture, and damaging chemicals. Respirators should be stored in such a manner as to retain their natural shape.[21]

Conclusion

As with the facility, an organization's staff can help contribute to an unsafe work environment. Organization leaders must put plans in place to address human factors related to safety as well as work together with employees to improve the overall safety of the environment. ■

References

1. CDC/NIOSH: Violence. *Occupational Hazards in Hospitals*, 2002.

2. Joint Commission Resources: *Security Issues for Today's Health Care Organization*. Oakbrook Terrace, IL: Joint Commission on Accreditation of Healthcare Organizations, 2002.

3. U.S. Department of Labor: Occupational Safety and Health Administration: *Guidelines for Preventing Workplace Violence for Health Care & Social Service Workers*, OSHA 3148-01R, 2004.

4. Joint Commission Resources: *Environment of Care Handbook, Second Edition*. Oakbrook Terrace, IL: Joint Commission on Accreditation of Healthcare Organizations, 2004.

5. Joint Commission Resources: Designing for security in the emergency department. *Environment of Care News:* 6: 11, Mar. 2003.

6. Department of Health and Human Services: *Current Intelligence Bulletin 57 Violence: Risk Factors and Prevention Strategies*, DHHS (NIOSH) Publication No. 96–100.

7. U.S. Department of Justice: National Crime Victimization Survey. http://www.ojp.usdoj.gov/bjs/cvict.htm (accessed Sep. 30, 2002).

8. Joint Commission Resources: A Violence Prevention Program for Worker Safety. *Environment of Care News* 8: 6, Jun. 2005.

9. U.S. Department of Labor: Occupational Safety and Health Administration: *Guidelines for Nursing Homes: Ergonomics for the Prevention of Musculoskeletal Disorders*. http://www.osha.gov/ergonomics/guidelines/nursinghome/final_nh_guidelines.html (accessed Mar. 19, 2005).

10. Joint Commission Resources: Back injuries among health care workers in acute care settings – part 1. *Environment of Care News* 7: 2-3, Jun. 2004.

11. Joint Commission Resources: Back injuries among health care workers in acute care settings – part 2. *Environment of Care News* 7: 10-11, Jul. 2004.

12. Interview with Audrey Nelson, Ph.D., R.N., F.A.A.N., director of the Veterans Administration (VA) Patient Safety Research Center, February 8, 2005.

13. U.S. Department of Labor: Occupational Safety and Health Administration: *Coverage and Definitions*. http://www.osha.gov/pls/oshaweb/owadisp.show_document?p_table=STANDARDS&p_id=12886 (accessed Mar. 19, 2005).

14. U.S. Department of Labor: Occupational Safety and Health Administration: *1910 Subpart E Appendix*. http://www.osha.gov/pls/oshaweb/owadisp.show_document?p_table=STANDARDS&p_id=10114 (accessed Mar. 19, 2005).

Chapter 3: Human Factor-Related Risks

15. U.S. Department of Labor: Occupational Safety and Health Administration: *How to Plan for Workplace Emergencies and Evacuations.* http://www.osha.gov/Publications/osha3088.pdf (accessed Feb. 10, 2005).

16. Joint Commission Resources: Gas Leak Emergency. *Environment of Care News* 7: 8-9, Apr. 2004.

17. U.S. Department of Labor, Occupational Safety and Health Administration: *Non-mandatory Compliance Guidelines for Hazard Assessment and Personal Protective Equipment Selection.* http://www.osha.gov/pls/oshaweb/owadisp.show_document?p_table=STANDARDS&p_id=10120 (accessed Mar. 19, 2005).

18. U.S. Department of Labor, Occupational Safety and Health Administration: *General Requirements.* http://www.osha.gov/pls/oshaweb/owadisp.show_document?p_table=STANDARDS&p_id=9777 (accessed Mar. 19, 2005).

19. U.S. Department of Labor: Occupational Safety and Health Administration: *Personal Protective Equipment.* http://www.osha.gov/Publications/osha3151.pdf (accessed Mar. 19, 2005).

20. Joint Commission Resources: Staying Safe in a Gastro Outbreak. *Environment of Care News* 8: 6-7 and 11, Apr. 2005.

21. U.S. Department of Labor: Occupational Safety and Health Administration: *Respiratory Protection.* http://www.osha.gov/Publications/osha3079.pdf (accessed Mar. 19, 2005).

22. Joint Commission Resources: A respiratory protection program for worker safety. *Environment of Care News* 8: 6-7, July, 2005.

23. U.S. Department of Labor: Occupational Safety and Health Administration: *Respiratory Protection e-Tool.* http://www.osha.gov/SLTC/etools/respiratory/index.html (accessed Mar. 19, 2005).

24. U.S. Department of Labor, Occupational Safety and Health Administration: *Respirator Medical Evaluation Questionnaire.* http://www.osha.gov/pls/oshaweb/owadisp.show_document?p_table=STANDARDS&p_id=9783 (accessed Mar. 19, 2005).

25. U.S. Department of Labor, Occupational Safety and Health Administration: *Respiratory Protection.* http://www.osha.gov/pls/oshaweb/owadisp.show_document?p_table=STANDARDS&p_id=12716 (accessed Mar. 19, 2005).

26. U.S. Department of Labor, Occupational Safety and Health Administration: *Fit Testing Procedures.* http://www.osha.gov/pls/oshaweb/owadisp.show_document?p_table=STANDARDS&p_id=9780 (accessed Mar. 19, 2005).

27. Association for Professionals in Infection Control and Epidemiology: Political moves. *APIC News* 23: Jan. 2005.

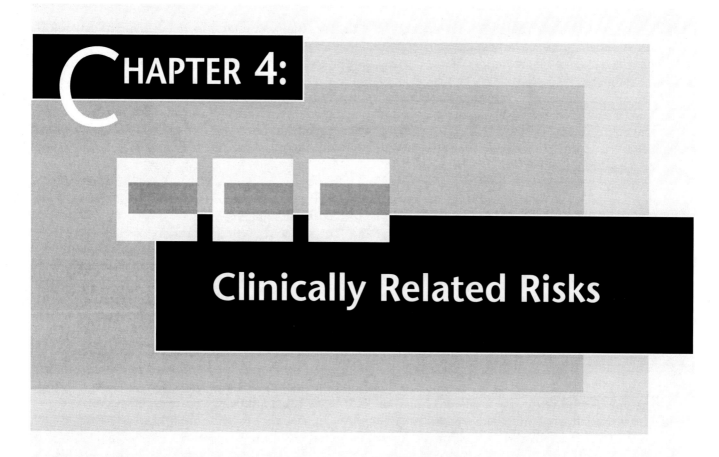

Chapter 4:

Clinically Related Risks

Worker safety in health care organizations is subject to some risks that are unique to the industry. For example, workers themselves may develop diseases brought into the organization by the individuals served. Tools used, such as needles and sutures, may be carriers of disease. Processes performed in a health care organization may involve chemicals or drugs that one would not likely be exposed to in another work environment.

Every occupation has its risks. Previous chapters of this book have addressed issues that cross a wide spectrum of industry, including health care. This chapter will address risks that are more prevalent in health care by the nature of the services provided. These risks may occur in other industries, but are probably more incidental in nature.

Topics addressed in this chapter include worker exposure to bloodborne pathogens and associated exposures; to diseases such as tuberculosis (TB) and *Legionella;* to chemicals, including ethylene oxide, formaldehyde, and glutaraldehyde; and to hazardous drugs and anesthetic gases.

BLOODBORNE PATHOGENS

OSHA defines bloodborne pathogens as "pathogenic microorganisms that are present in human blood and can cause disease in humans."[1] In practice, the definition is expanded to include those pathogens present not only in blood, but in other potentially infectious materials, such as other body fluids. Bloodborne pathogens (BBP) include most notably HIV and hepatitis B and C; these pose the greatest risk to workers.

Standards and Requirements

The Joint Commission addresses the issue of bloodborne pathogens under EC.3.10, which discusses hazardous materials and waste management. In a footnote to the standard itself, hazardous materials and waste are defined as "materials whose handling, use, and storage are guided or regulated by local, state, or federal regulation." The footnote goes on to state, "Examples include OSHA's Regulations for Bloodborne Pathogens (regarding the blood, other infectious materials, contaminated items which would release blood or other infectious materials, or contaminated sharps)."

Of course the effective management of an environmental health and safety program as required under EC.1.10 is the overarching rule. Without that, it would be difficult to comply with the rest of the standards. Training and education requirements related to bloodborne pathogens are found in the Human Resources chapter at HR.2.10, HR.2.20, and HR.2.30.

STANDARDS — Joint Commission Standards that Address Bloodborne Pathogens

- EC.1.10, Safety Management; EC.1.20, Environmental Tours; EC.3.10, Hazardous Materials & Waste Management; EC.9.10, Monitoring Environmental Conditions; EC.9.20, Analyzing Environmental Issues; EC.9.30, Improving the Environment
- HR.2.10, Initial Job Training; HR.2.20, Roles & Responsibilities; HR.2.30, Ongoing Education

OSHA's Bloodborne Pathogen Standard is found at 29CFR 1910.1030. It was first issued by OSHA in 1991 to protect workers from the risk of exposure to pathogens through contact with blood and body fluids. This was a time when the AIDS epidemic was on the rise. Ten years later, the Needlestick Safety and Prevention Act was passed by the U.S. Congress in an effort to further reduce exposure, and OSHA updated its BBP standard in response.

OSHA's standard is especially applicable to health care organizations and regulates exposure to blood and body fluids (which can include unfixed tissues or organs, and cultures) via any method, including splashes, spills, puncture wounds, and so forth. This standard requires an exposure control plan, appropriate engineering controls (including protected needle devices and sharps disposal containers), personal protective equipment (PPE), labeling, and disposal. Reporting mechanisms and programs of prophylaxis must be in place for any individuals who do become exposed. Annual orientation and education is specified for individuals who may reasonably be expected to be exposed to blood and body fluids in the course of performing their job duties.[2] The following sections make reference to the OSHA requirements, but for a comprehensive listing, please see OSHA's Web site at http://www.osha.gov.

Hazards and Exposure

Bloodborne pathogen hazards abound in a health care setting. As already noted, the three pathogens that get the most attention are HIV and hepatitis B and C. These are diseases that can be devastating, if not fatal, to an employee or patient who contracts them. Other infectious agents that can be transmitted through blood and body fluids include hepatitis A, staphylococcus and Streptococcus infections, Salmonella and/or Shigella-induced gastroenteritis, pneumonia, syphilis, malaria, measles, and the list goes on.

Pathogens are found in other areas in addition to blood. Figure 4-1 contains a listing of potentially infectious materials other than blood.

The possibilities for exposure to bloodborne pathogens are numerous. Worker exposure results when the potentially infectious material comes in contact with an open wound, non-intact skin (chapped or scraped), or mucous membranes, such as in the nose or mouth, or around the eyes.

Many activities of necessity in a healthcare organization require direct contact with blood and body fluids. For example, splashes can occur in surgical settings, while treating wounds, during dressing changes, opening tubes of blood, discarding potentially infectious medical waste, and many other activities.

Needlestick injuries, where the worker's skin is pierced by a contaminated needle, are among the most frequently experienced exposures and are a cause of great concern in health care organizations. Needle usage is present in phlebotomy activities, starting IVs, performing sutures, and so forth. Much emphasis has been placed on the risks of needlesticks and other sharps injuries for clinical staff. However, environmental services employees, including housekeepers, sanitation workers, and laundry workers are often the recipients of sharps injuries.[3]

Further complicating the issue is that staff may not know which individual or which tube of blood contains a bloodborne pathogen. Patient privacy regulations play a large part in this, but one must not forget that in some cases, the disease is not yet diagnosed. Therefore all patients and all specimens must be considered potentially infectious.

Exposure Control Plan

A bloodborne pathogens (BBP) exposure control plan is the organization's written program to reduce or eliminate employees' exposure to bloodborne pathogens. OSHA requires organizations to create and implement such a plan. While the Joint Commission does not require compliance with OSHA regulations, the concept of an exposure control plan is a good one and merits organizational consideration.

Chapter 4: Clinically Related Risks

Figure 4-1. Other Potentially Infectious Materials[1]

Semen	Saliva in dental procedures
Vaginal secretions	Any body fluid visibly contaminated with blood
Cerebrospinal fluid	All body fluids in situations where it is difficult or impossible to differentiate between body fluids
Synovial fluid	Any unfixed human tissue or organ
Pleural fluid	HIV-containing cell, tissue, or organ cultures
Pericardial fluid	HIV- or HBV-containing culture medium
Peritoneal fluid	Blood, organs, or tissues from experimental animals infected with HIV or HBV
Amniotic fluid	

Blood is not the only concern in protecting against infectious exposure.
Source: U.S. Department of Labor, Occupational Safety and Health Administration.

According to OSHA, the exposure control plan must be available to all employees and must be reviewed and updated as often as necessary, but at least annually. Revisions must reflect any changes in technology that have occurred in the interim that may eliminate or reduce BBP exposure. Revisions must also include any safer medical devices that have been evaluated and considered.

Exposure Determination
OSHA defines "occupational exposure" as "reasonably anticipated skin, eye, mucous membrane, or parenteral* contact with blood or other potentially infectious materials that may result from the performance of an employee's duties." Based on this definition, employers should determine in which jobs all employees, or some employees, have occupational exposure. If only some of the employees in a particular job classification perform duties with occupational exposure, then a list of specific duties or tasks that result in exposure should be developed to indicate which employees are at risk. If all employees in a job classification are potentially exposed, than no such list is necessary.

Controls
One important control that organizations can use to address bloodborne pathogens exposure is *Standard Precautions* (previously called Universal Precautions). This means treating all blood and other potentially infectious materials as if they were infectious. Standard precautions involve using gloves, face protection, and gowns as well as developing engineering and work practice controls to avoid exposure.

Engineering and Work Practice Controls.
As mentioned previously in this publication, engineering and work practice controls are preferable to PPE. PPE should be used when exposure remains after the implementation of higher-level controls. According to OSHA, engineering controls for bloodborne pathogens "isolate or remove the bloodborne pathogens hazard from the workplace and may include sharps disposal containers, self-sheathing needles, and needleless systems."[1] See Figure 4-2 on page 90 for definitions of some of these controls.

Safer Needle Devices
Safer needle devices have certain features including the following:
- Following use, a barrier is provided between the needle and the user's hands
- The user's hands are behind the needle at all times
- The device is an integral component of the needle or system, and not an accessory
- Protection is provided before, during, and after use and disposal
- Safety features are simple and intuitive, with little need for training or expertise[5]

Although no specific types of safer needle devices are mandated by the Joint Commission or OSHA, OSHA does mandate that organizations continually reevaluate their prevention program and investigate any new technology that may become available, with the intent of driving the needlestick injury rate as low as possible.

The sidebar on page 91 provides some suggestions that may help organizations select and evaluate needle devices.

---
* According to OSHA, "Parenteral" is defined as "piercing mucous membranes or the skin barrier through such events as needlesticks, human bites, cuts, and abrasions."

> ### ▪▪▪ Figure 4-2. Engineering Controls[4]
>
> A number of engineering controls can be used to prevent sharps injuries.
>
> **Sharps with Engineered Sharps Injury Protections**
>
> These include non-needle sharps or needle devices containing built-in safety features that are used for collecting fluids or administering medications or other fluids, or other procedures involving the risk of sharps injury. This description covers a broad array of devices, including:
>
> - Syringes with a sliding sheath that shields the attached needle after use
> - Needles that retract into a syringe after use
> - Shielded or retracting catheters
> - Intravenous medication (IV) delivery systems that use a catheter port with a needle housed in a protective covering
>
> **Needleless Systems**
>
> These are devices that provide an alternative to needles for various procedures to reduce the risk of injury involving contaminated sharps. Examples include:
>
> - IV medication systems that administer medication or fluids through a catheter port using non-needle connections
> - jet injection systems that deliver liquid medication beneath the skin or through a muscle
>
> *Sharps injuries can be prevented by engineering controls, among other cautions.*
>
> **Source:** U.S. Department of Labor, Occupational Safety and Health Administration.

Engineering and work practice controls must be implemented with respect to the handling of contaminated sharps. A policy prohibiting the recapping, removing, or bending of contaminated needles or other sharps must be in place and in force, unless the employer can demonstrate that there is no viable alternative. Breaking contaminated needles is prohibited under all circumstances.

Sharps disposal containers are mandated to be puncture resistant, labeled or color coded, and leakproof. They must be easily accessible and as close as possible to the area where sharps are used. The containers must not be allowed to overfill and they must be replaced on a regular basis. When picked up for removal or otherwise moved, they must be closed to prevent spillage or any other exposure to the sharps. Reusable sharps are rare today, but if used, under no circumstance should an employee have to retrieve them by reaching in a sharps disposal container.

In addition to the handling of contaminated sharps, organizations must have policies in place to prevent exposure to BBPs through other methods. For example, the Joint Commission and OSHA require organizations to have hand washing facilities available and accessible to staff, or if that is not feasible, other antiseptic hand cleanser must be provided. Employees must wash their hands as soon as possible after removing gloves or other PPE. If an employee has had contact with blood or body fluids, hands or skin must be washed with soap and water as soon as possible. If the contact is with a mucous membrane, that area should be flushed with water immediately after contact.

In addition to handwashing, procedures should be developed to address the following exposure scenarios:
- Eating, drinking, smoking, applying cosmetics or lip balm, and handling contact lenses in a work area with reasonably anticipated exposure
- Food and drink in refrigerators, freezers, shelves, cabinets, countertops, or bench tops where blood or OPIM (other potentially infectious materials) are present
- Mouth pipetting or suctioning blood or OPIM
- PPE worn outside the work area

TIP ▶ Most heath care organizations do have these policies in place, but many times they are not practiced and enforced. One of the most frequently seen infractions is food and beverages in areas where blood and OPIM are present.

Equipment that may become contaminated with blood or OPIM during use must be checked and decontaminated, if necessary and feasible, prior to shipment or servicing. It must be tagged with a biohazard label that states which portion of the machine remains contaminated, and this information must be communicated to affected employees or servicing representatives.

Chapter 4: Clinically Related Risks

Nonmanagerial staff members who are involved in direct patient care should have input into the evaluation and selection of engineering and work practice controls to reduce or eliminate BBP exposure. Participating employees should reflect a range of exposure situations and multiple departments. OSHA requires employers to document how they received employee input in the exposure control plan.

Personal Protective Equipment

Employers are required to provide to the employee, free of charge, any appropriate PPE where occupational exposure occurs. OSHA states that PPE is "appropriate" "only if it does not permit blood or other potentially infectious materials to pass through to or reach the employee's work clothes, street clothes, undergarments, skin, eyes, mouth, or other mucous membranes under normal conditions of use and for the duration of time which the protective equipment will be used."[1]

Additional employer responsibilities with respect to PPE include providing appropriate sizes and ready accessibility. If an employee is allergic to the latex in gloves, for example, an alternate choice must be made available. If repairs or replacements are needed, they must be employer-provided. Any mandated PPE must be cleaned, laundered, and disposed of by the employer.

Under OSHA regulations, the use of employer-provided PPE is mandatory; however, there is an exception for "rare and extraordinary circumstances" when an employee judges that the use of the PPE would hinder the delivery of health care services or would pose a safety hazard. These circumstances should be investigated and documented.

PPE is discussed in further detail in Chapter Three, but the following is a brief discussion of PPE that specifically helps prevent exposure to bloodborne pathogens.

Gloves should be worn for reasonably anticipated hand exposure to blood or OPIM, mucous membranes, or non-intact skin. Employees should wear gloves when conducting vascular access procedures (phlebotomies, starting IVs, and so forth) and gloves should also be used when touching contaminated items or surfaces. Gloves should be changed as soon as possible after they become contaminated, or if they are torn, punctured, or otherwise compromised.

Eye masks, goggles, and face shields are just some of the types of PPE employees can use to prevent splashes to the face. Such equipment should be worn when splashing is reasonably anticipated.

Sidebar 4-1. Selecting Safer Needle Devices

1. Identify priorities and prevention strategies. Look at your needlestick- and sharps-related injury reports to determine the devices most commonly involved, how injuries occur and in what areas, and the types of workers who are most often affected. Local and national Web sites, such as those maintained by the CDC and OSHA, provide information about devices and work practices that have helped others reduce injuries.

2. Replace needle devices whenever possible. Eliminating any unnecessary use of needles and using devices with safety features are significant components of your prevention program. A few examples of available alternatives to traditional needle devices include needleless IV delivery systems; needles that retract into a syringe or vacuum tube holder; and hinged or sliding shields attached to phlebotomy needles, winged-steel needles, and blood gas needles

3. Review and modify work practices. Even though certain procedures have been shown to increase the risk for needlesticks, many are still practiced regularly. Elimination of manual recapping, proper disposal of needles and sharps, and a specimen collection process that reduces the number of times needles are used on a patient can all help reduce the risk of injuries.

4. Train employees. Having safer devices and establishing better practices are useless unless health care workers receive training in their proper use and implement them across your organization, respectively. Part of your safety training program can promote the importance of all employees being alert to the dangers of exposed needles and sharps—not just to themselves but to patients.

5. Report needlesticks and injuries. The CDC estimates that almost half of all needlesticks go unreported. Encourage workers to report all needlesticks and injuries related to sharps to ensure that they receive appropriate follow-up care. Complete records of where and how injuries have occurred are also vital to identifying and prioritizing high-risk areas to be addressed in your organization.[6]

Protective body clothing includes gowns, aprons, and lab coats. The proper material for this clothing depends on the type of exposure. Surgical caps and shoe covers must be worn when gross contamination can be anticipated. It is important in these circumstances to emphasize the fact that this PPE may not be worn outside the work area.

Housekeeping, Waste, and Laundry

Work practice controls should be used when handling spills, waste disposal, and laundry processes. Countertops and other work surfaces must be disinfected as soon as possible after a spill or when they are overtly contaminated. As a matter of routine, such surfaces should be decontaminated at the end of a work shift. If protective coverings are used on work surfaces or equipment, they should be changed when they become contaminated, and at the end of the work shift.

Regulated waste is defined as "liquid or semi-liquid blood or other potentially infectious materials; contaminated items that would release blood or other potentially infectious materials in a liquid or semi-liquid state if compressed; items that are caked with dried blood or other potentially infectious materials that are capable of releasing these materials during handling; contaminated sharps; and pathological and microbiological wastes containing blood or other potentially infectious materials."[1] Containers for regulated waste should have similar characteristics to those for contaminated sharps. They should be closable, constructed to contain all contents and prevent leakage, appropriately labeled or color coded, and closed prior to removal to prevent spillage or protrusion of contents. Disposal of regulated medical waste is in accordance with applicable law and regulation.

Laundry that has been contaminated may include patient gowns, sheets, towels, and drapes that have been used by patients. In addition, laundry may include employer-provided PPE, such as lab coats and surgical scrubs that have become soiled. Contaminated laundry must be placed in bags or containers labeled or color coded as biohazardous. Under standard precautions, when all laundry is treated as potentially contaminated, alternate labeling or color coding is acceptable if it is recognizable by all employees. If the laundry is contaminated to the degree that it may soak through a laundry bag or leak from a container, it must be placed in a container that will prevent leakage. Note that laundry employees must be provided with appropriate PPE.

Hepatitis B Vaccination

All job classifications and/or employees who have been determined to have occupational exposure to pathogens should be designated to receive the hepatitis B vaccination series. According to OSHA requirements, the vaccine must be made available to all employees with potential occupational exposure within 10 days of their initial assignment to the work area. Exceptions are when the employee has previously received the hepatitis B vaccination series, antibody testing demonstrates employee immunity, or there are medical contraindications to vaccination.

Employees who have potential occupational exposure may, however, decline the vaccination. If they originally decline, and change their mind at a latter date, the vaccine should be provided at that time. If they choose to decline the vaccination series, they must sign a declination statement. OSHA has specific requirements as to the content of that statement, contained in Appendix A of the Bloodborne Pathogens Standard. Organizations should check the OSHA Web site (http://www.osha.gov) for the exact content.

After the vaccination series is completed, employees should be tested for antibodies. Organizations should refer to the CDC's guidelines regarding antibody testing. The guidelines state that healthcare workers "who have contact with patients or blood and are at ongoing risk for percutaneous injuries should be tested 1-2 months after completion of the 3-dose vaccination series for anti-HBs (antibody to hepatitis B, which would be expected to develop in a vaccinated individual). Persons who do not respond to the primary vaccine series should complete a second 3-dose vaccine series or be evaluated to determine if they are HBs-Ag positive (a carrier of the hepatitis B antigen). Re-vaccinated persons should be retested at the completion of the second vaccine series." If an employee still does not test positive for the antibody, a third series of vaccinations need not be given.[7]

Employee Exposure

If an employee is exposed to blood or other potentially infectious materials in a manner that may transmit disease, the health care organization should provide a confidential medical examination and appropriate follow-up care. OSHA has specific requirements regarding the content of this medical examination, including the following:

- Documentation of the exposure route and circumstances
- Identification of the source individual, unless prohibited by law or it is not feasible
- Blood testing of the source individual (with consent) to determine HIV and HBV status (unless previously known)
- Results of the source individual testing made known to the exposed employee
- Determination of employee's HIV and HBV serological status
- Post-exposure prophylaxis as indicated
- Counseling and evaluation of any reported illness

According to OSHA requirements, the physician evaluating an employee exposure must be provided with a copy of OSHA's Bloodborne Pathogens Standard, a description of the employee's duties, circumstances and route of exposure, the source individual's blood testing results, and the relevant employee's medical records. A written opinion must be provided that reflects only whether hepatitis B vaccination is indicated and whether or not the employee has received it. In addition, the opinion must state that the employee has been informed of the results of the evaluation and any medical conditions that may require evaluation or treatment.

Medical records should be established by the employer for all employees who have received an exposure. These records should be kept confidential and not disclosed without the employee's consent. OSHA requires such medical records to be kept for the duration of employment plus 30 years. Content of the records will include a copy of the employee's HBV vaccination status, a copy of examination results, a copy of the health care professional's written opinion, and a copy of the information provided to the health care professional.

OSHA also requires a sharps injury log to be maintained by the employer to record all percutaneous injuries from contaminated sharps. The device involved must be identified by brand and type. The work area of the incident must be recorded, along with an explanation of how the incident occurred. This log must be kept to ensure the confidentiality of the injured employee. Please see Chapter One for more information on OSHA recordkeeping and the OSHA 300 log.

Training

All employees with potential occupational exposure should participate in a training program at the time of their initial assignment to the tasks with potential exposure and at least annually thereafter. Additional training should be provided when there is a change to the tasks or procedures related to the occupational exposure. Contents of the training program must include:

- An accessible copy of the OSHA's Bloodborne Pathogens Standard
- An explanation of its contents
- Epidemiology and symptoms of bloodborne disease
- Modes of transmission of bloodborne pathogens
- The organization's exposure control plan and how the employee can obtain a copy
- How to recognize potential exposures
- How to limit potential exposure through various levels of controls
- Types, use, location, removal, handling, decontamination, and disposal of PPE
- Basis for selection of PPE
- Information on the HBV vaccine, including efficacy, safety, administration, benefits, and that it is offered at no charge to the employee
- Who to contact in an emergency situation involving blood or OPIM
- Procedure to follow in the event of an exposure
- Post-exposure evaluation
- Signs, labels, and color coding

An opportunity for interactive questions and answers must be available to the employees. This can be met in one of several ways, the most obvious being a live training session. Computer-based training and videotaped training are permissible, but someone must still be available to answer questions. If this individual is not available in person, he or she may be contacted electronically (via phone, fax, or e-mail), but this must take place in real time. According to OSHA requirements, training records must contain the date(s) of the session(s), the contents or a summary thereof, the names and qualifications of the trainer(s), and the names and job titles of the attendees. Training records must be kept for three years following the training date.

Tuberculosis

Mycobacterium tuberculosis (M. tuberculosis), the bacterium that causes TB, is carried through the air in particles called *droplet nuclei*. It is not transmitted by surface contact. If these droplet nuclei are inhaled, infection can occur in a susceptible individual. The probability that an exposed individual will become infected is proportional to the concentration of the droplet nuclei in the air and the length of exposure.

The number of cases of TB in the United States was in a steady decline until 1985. Starting the following year, the rate began to climb, and with it came a resurgence of interest in this disease and its control. In addition, drug-resistant strains of the disease were identified.

In 1993, the incidence of TB again began to decline. This trend continued following the issuance of CDC guidelines in 1994 and their adoption by health care organizations.

Despite the recent decline in incidence, TB remains a deadly disease compounded by an increase in the number of immunosuppressed individuals—such as those who are HIV infected—in the population. In 2003, the CDC reported 14,874 cases.[8] With these facts and statistics as a backdrop, this section will address TB-related regulation and control within health care organizations today.

Standards and Regulations

Several Joint Commission standards relate to worker protection from exposure to TB. The first is the general requirement in EC.1.10 for an effective environmental health and safety program. Second, the utilities management standard, EC.7.10, requires organizations to reduce the potential for organization-acquired illness such as TB to be transmitted through the utility systems. The standards require organizations to design, install, and maintain ventilation equipment to provide appropriate pressure relationships, air exchange rates, and filtration efficiencies for ventilation systems serving areas specially designed to control airborne contaminants such as Mycobacterium tuberculosis. In addition to the EC standards, the IC standards address the prevention and control of infection including TB (see standards callout). All these standards taken together emphasize the need for environment of care professionals to work with infection control professionals on the prevention of exposure to TB, and have a particular bearing on the TB risk assessment process, discussed subsequently.

STANDARDS *Joint Commission Standards that Implicitly Address TB*

- ► EC.1.10, Safety Management; EC.1.20, Environmental Tours; EC.3.10, Hazardous Materials & Waste Management; EC.7.10, Utilities Management (EP16); EC.9.10, Monitoring Environmental Conditions; EC.9.20, Analyzing Environmental Issues; EC.9.30, Improving the Environment
- ► IC.2.10, Identifying Risks (EP1, EP2, EP3); IC.3.10, Establishing Priorities (EP2); IC.4.10, Implementing Strategies (EP1)
- ► HR.2.10, Initial Job Training; HR.2.20, Roles & Responsibilities; HR.2.30, Ongoing Education

---

OSHA Requirements

OSHA issued a proposed comprehensive standard covering occupational exposure to TB in 1997. In 2003, OSHA ceased work on the standard. However, OSHA continues to be involved in efforts to decrease this workplace hazard through enforcement efforts as well as educational and collaborative strategies. Enforcement involves several OSHA standards (for example, 29CFR 1910.1020, Access to Employee Exposure and Medical Records; 29CFR 1910.134, Respiratory Protection; 29CFR 1910.132, Personal Protective Equipment General Requirements) as well as Section 5(a)(1), the general duty clause, of the Occupational Safety and Health Act for compliance with CDC Guidelines. See http://www.osha.gov for more information about current OSHA efforts regarding TB in the workplace.

CDC Guidelines

In 1994, the CDC first released their guidelines regarding the transmission of TB in health care facilities. At the time of this writing, the 1994 guidelines are still in effect, but a draft of a proposed 2005 revision is open for comment. Because this latter document is only in draft format, the exact requirements will not be known until the revision is published in its final form. Discussion of this proposal will be limited to general directions that will most likely be taken with the new document.

In the overview to the 2005 draft guidelines, the rationale for the update includes advances in science and practice. The revised guidelines "place emphasis on actions to maintain momentum and expertise needed to avert another TB resurgence and to eliminate the lingering threat to health care workers, which is mainly from patients or others with unsuspected and undiagnosed infectious TB disease."[9] The revision will address a broader section of health care settings, to include inpatient, outpatient, and nontraditional settings, such as emergency medical services, home health care, laboratories, and so forth. The 1994 edition is primarily aimed at hospitals.

Some of the proposed changes from the 1994 guidelines include the following:
- More aspects of infection control considered in the risk assessment
- In some settings, a reduced frequency of TB screening
- Guideline applicability to an entire setting instead of specific areas
- Revised recommendations for annual respirator training and user seal-checking
- Expanded information on ultraviolet germicidal irradiation (UVGI) and room air recirculation

The CDC guidelines provide detailed requirements that organizations must meet. These requirements form the basis of the discussion in the following sections.

Chapter 4: Clinically Related Risks

Hazards

Although the incidence of TB is declining, health care workers remain at risk of exposure. According to the CDC, health care and long-term care facilities are the highest risk work places. Still, the Society for Healthcare Epidemiologists of America (SHEA) notes that health care workers "represent a small proportion of all cases and are not disproportionately represented in the TB caseload compared to their presence in the workforce."[10]

Many times transmission of TB in the workplace happens when workers do not realize that a patient has infectious TB. Data from the Association for Professionals in Infection Control and Epidemiology (APIC), show that 75.6% of health care workers infected in TB outbreaks since 1960 were from an "undiagnosed and unsuspected TB patient."[10] Geographic variation in the incidence of TB must also be noted, , ranging from a low of 0.9 cases per 100,000 population in North Dakota to a high of 9.0 per 100,000 in California.[9] Health care workers therefore face different levels of risk in different parts of the country. All these facts taken together highlight the importance of maintaining an index of suspicion for TB and appropriately isolating any suspected or confirmed cases.

A TB Prevention and Control Program

A program to control TB exposure in a health care organization is one part of an effective infection control program. To avoid the exposure of workers to unidentified cases, early identification and isolation of suspected individuals are critical. Policies and procedures must be in place, reviewed periodically, and monitored for effectiveness.

The CDC recommends the following to reduce the risk of TB transmission:

- Assigning supervisory responsibility for the TB infection control program
- Conducting a risk assessment
- Developing a program based on the risk assessment
- Developing, implementing, and enforcing policies and protocols for early identification, evaluation, and treatment
- Prompt triage for potential TB patients in outpatient settings
- Promptly initiating and maintaining isolation for suspected inpatient cases
- Effective discharge planning
- Developing and maintaining engineering controls, such as ventilation (see the "Controls" section later in this chapter)
- Developing and implementing a respiratory protection program
- Using precautions for cough-inducing procedures
- Training and education for staff
- Implementing a program of periodic counseling and TB screening for staff
- Evaluating potential TB outbreaks, including skin test conversions for health care workers
- Coordination with the public health department[11]

Responsibility

The Joint Commission infection control standard, IC.7.10, requires effective management of an infection control program in a health care organization. The responsibility may be managed by one individual or a group, "whose number, competency, and skill mix are determined by the goals and objectives of the IC activities." The qualifications of these individuals are again based on the identified risks, the patient population and the complexity of the anticipated activities, and these qualifications may be achieved through education, training, experience, or certification.

Risk Assessment

The CDC 1994 guidelines call for a risk assessment for the transmission of TB for the entire facility, with area-specific assessments as needed in locations such as the emergency department, pulmonary clinics, and inpatient settings as appropriate. Suggested participants include specialists in epidemiology, infectious disease, and/or pulmonary disease, infection control practitioners, health care administrators, occupational health staff, engineers, or local public health personnel. Ultimately the health care organization must decide who should be involved, but clinical input is essential.

The profile of TB in the community should be examined via public health records, along with any records of TB cases in the health care organization. If there are no cases in either population, then the organization may classify itself as having minimal risk.

If documented cases exist, then the records of health care worker screening should be examined to determine if there is a higher conversion rate on the PPD testing in certain areas or any evidence of person-to-person transmission. If this assessment proves to be negative, classification can be determined as follows:

- Very low risk: No TB patients admitted to the **facility** as inpatients during preceding year and plan to refer patients with confirmed or suspected TB to another facility if inpatient care is required.

- Low risk: Fewer than six TB patients admitted to the **area** during the preceding year.
- Intermediate risk: Six or more TB patients admitted to the **area** during the preceding year.

If the assessment of health care worker screening did show higher rates or clusters of conversion or evidence of interpersonal transmission, then the causes of transmission must be evaluated. If the causes have been rectified, and repeat testing among staff shows no further conversions or transmission, than choose the appropriate level of risk from the above grouping. If the causes of transmission have not been identified and corrected or if subsequent evidence of staff seroconversion or transmission arises, then the facility is at high risk.[11]

Based on the outcome of this risk assessment process, organizations should develop a plan for addressing TB infection control. Such a plan should be implemented as indicated for each area of the facility. Areas where cough-inducing protocols are performed should be considered to be at intermediate risk. The implementation of the protocols should be monitored periodically, with more frequent monitoring being performed in higher-risk areas. Risk assessments should also be repeated periodically at an interval dependent on the level of risk.

Staff Testing

Based on the risk assessment, health care workers who could potentially be exposed to TB should participate in a screening program for latent TB. The CDC recommends baseline testing for individuals in all risk categories except minimal, where testing is optional.

Routine periodic screening is not applicable for those with minimal risk. In very low-risk facilities, the recommendation is variable dependent on the duties of the staff member; however, those who work in areas where patients are diagnosed and admitted would benefit from routine periodic screening. Staff members who work in low-risk areas should be screened on an annual basis, but those in intermediate areas should be screened every 6 to 12 months. Those in high-risk areas should be screened quarterly. Physicians and other contracted workers who are not employees should also be tested according to the risk assessment for their work area.

Screening of health care workers for latent TB is important to prevent the spread of TB to others. Any employees who have a positive skin test or who convert to a positive test after previous negatives must receive appropriate counseling and therapy. Not all these positive tests are the result of workplace exposure, and an investigation should be done to verify any potential outside source before concluding work relatedness.

Controls

The CDC recommends that organizations use engineering, administrative and work practice, and PPE controls to reduce the risk of TB exposure and transmission. Administrative controls impact the largest number of people. They are intended to reduce the risk of exposing those who are not infected. Examples of administrative controls include:

- Policies and protocols for prompt identification, evaluation, isolation, and treatment of suspected cases
- Procedures for effective work practices such as respiratory protection and closing doors to isolation rooms
- A program to screen health care workers for TB infection, as described above.

Engineering controls are intended to prevent the spread of droplet nuclei through effective use of the heating, ventilating, and air conditioning (HVAC) system and other engineered devices. One such engineering control is the isolation room. Isolation rooms, now termed "airborne infectious isolation," or AII, should be private rooms specially equipped to contain the droplet nuclei within the room and reduce their concentration through appropriate ventilation design. AIIs must be maintained under negative pressure to prevent the droplet nuclei from entering the corridor, and the doors must be closed at all times. While a patient stays in the AII room, the negative pressure should be monitored daily, using a mechanical indicator or smoke tubes to ensure appropriate direction of air flow.

Current recommendations for air exchange rates in health care facilities, based on the American Society of Heating, Refrigerating, and Air-Conditioning Engineers (ASHRAE) and the American Institute of Architects (AIA) recommendations, are for six air changes per hour. This is based on comfort and odor control. To reduce the concentration of droplet nuclei in AII rooms, 12 or more air changes per hour are recommended where feasible. New construction or renovation should be designed to meet this recommendation.

AII rooms should be exhausted directly to the outside, and not recirculated within the facility. This is not always possible, however, and if not, high-efficiency particulate air (HEPA) filters should be installed in the room's exhaust duct to remove particles and infectious bacteria before they are introduced into the general ventilation. (The 2005 draft guidelines mandate HEPA filtration when discharging air from an AII room into the general ventilation.) HEPA filtration should also be used with local exhaust ventilation, such as used for booths for cough-producing and aerosol-generating procedures.

Other applications include use in portable air cleaners or fixed recirculation systems, where air is recirculated within an individual room.

Anterooms are not required for the AII room, but if provided, the pressure gradient should be positive relative to the room itself. Ultraviolet germicidal irradiation (UVGI) may be used at the upper level of the isolation room. It irradiates the upper air, adding to the effective air exchange rate and reducing the concentration of droplet nuclei. These units may be installed in a room, in a corridor, or in air ducts, but may not be used in place of HEPA filtration in air ducts discharging to general ventilation. Appropriate maintenance of UVGI systems includes monitoring the irradiance levels and changing the UV tubes as recommended or indicated. (The proposed 2005 draft guidelines offer additional information on UVGI.)

The number of AII rooms provided in a health care organization should be sufficient to accommodate the expected number of inpatients based on the risk assessment. Unless the organization is classified as minimal or very low risk, at least one AII room should be available. Both the 1994 and the proposed 2005 versions of the CDC's guidelines recommend grouping these rooms together to decrease the likelihood of transmitting TB and to facilitate the maintenance of optimal engineering controls. In addition, this configuration could be useful in an outbreak of infectious disease, such as might be seen in an incident of bioagent release.

PPE controls appropriate for TB include respiratory protection for all staff members who must enter a room with an individual with suspected or confirmed TB. An associated work practice control would be to reduce the number of individuals who must enter a room with a suspected or confirmed TB patient.

Training

Both the Joint Commission and the CDC require appropriate training regarding TB based on the occupational group and its risk for exposure. The following are components of a training program:[11]

- Basic concepts of *M. tuberculosis* transmission and disease
- Difference between latent infection and active disease; signs and symptoms
- Potential for occupational exposure
- Facility arrangements for appropriate isolation
- Infection control principles and practices to reduce risk, including hierarchy of controls
- Purpose of TB skin testing and significance of a positive result
- Preventive therapy for latent TB infection
- The worker's responsibility to seek prompt medical attention based on a positive test or symptoms and notify the health care organization
- Principles of drug therapy
- Confidentiality for the exposed worker
- Elevated risks due to immunosuppression
- Voluntary work reassignment for immunocompromised employees

Training should be provided before initial assignment to the work area, and repeated periodically, preferably annually.

LEGIONELLA

Legionella pneumophilia is the name of the bacterium that cause two related diseases, Legionnaires' Disease and Pontiac Fever. Many species of the bacteria have been identified. Legionellosis is the name of the infection, which can take either of the two forms.

At the 1976 American Legion Convention in Philadelphia, an outbreak of pneumonia resulted in 34 deaths. This first identification led to the name "Legionnaires' Disease," and subsequently to the name of the bacterium when it was identified by the CDC the following year. This is the more serious form of Legionellosis. This is the disease form that is contracted by the more susceptible individuals exposed to the bacteria, such as those middle aged and older, smokers, those with chronic lung disease, or those who are HIV positive or otherwise immunocompromised. It has an incubation period of 2 to 10 days.

Legionnaires' Disease affects between 8,000 and 18,000 people in the United States on an annual basis. Usually these are isolated cases not linked to an identified outbreak. Death occurs in 5% to 30% of the cases. Diagnosis depends on specialized testing; many cases of Legionnaires' Disease may be misdiagnosed as pneumonia, and are therefore unreported.[12]

A less serious form of Legionellosis is Pontiac Fever. It is not a pneumonia, and has more flu-like symptoms. Of the individuals who are not immunosuppressed, 90% or more of those exposed to *Legionella* contract this form of the disease, including otherwise healthy health care workers. The incubation period is usually one or two days, with recovery in two to five days.[12]

Legionella grows in water. Documented outbreaks have occurred when groups of individuals have breathed in aerosols from contaminated water sources in a variety of buildings including hospitals.

Standards and Requirements

Just as with TB, a number of Joint Commission standards relate to control of *Legionnella* in health care organizations. Again, EC.1.10 lays the foundation with requirements for an effective environmental health and safety program. EC.7.10 EP15 has particular bearing on the issue. "The organization identifies and implements processes to minimize pathogenic biological agents in cooling towers, domestic hot/cold water systems, and other aerosolizing water systems." Although this requirement can and does relate to other waterborne pathogens, *Legionella* is the agent of primary concern. (The standard is only applicable to hospital, long term care, and ambulatory care organizations.) As with TB, the infection control standards also relate to the prevention of exposure to *Legionella*.

STANDARDS — *Joint Commission Standards that Address Legionella*

➤ EC.1.10, Safety Management; EC.1.20, Environmental Tours; EC.3.10, Hazardous Materials & Waste Management; EC.7.10, Utilities Management (EP16); EC.9.10, Monitoring Environmental Conditions; EC.9.20, Analyzing Environmental Issues; EC.9.30, Improving the Environment;
➤ HR.2.10, Initial Job Training; HR.2.20, Roles & Responsibilities; HR.2.30, Ongoing Education

---

Although there is no OSHA regulation for *Legionella*, "safe and healthful working conditions" of the OSHA document include maintenance of water facilities and other places where *Legionella* or other pathogenic organisms can flourish. OSHA provides instructions for inspectors in its Technical Manual, Section III, Chapter 7.[13] The focus of these instructions is the prevention and control of potentially contaminated water sources rather than the identification of cases, although the instructions also provide a significant amount of information about the disease and testing.

Hazard

Legionella is common in all aquatic environments, both internal and external. It thrives on scale and biofilm in pipes and at the bottom of storage tanks, and it loves stagnant water. It favors water at 80° - 120°F, the temperature frequently found in plumbing systems, hot water tanks, cooling towers, and so forth. Dead legs in the plumbing system, or portions of the system that have been shut down, provide an excellent location for *Legionella* growth. Health care organizations report up to 1,300 cases of waterborne *Legionella pneumophilia* each year.

Common sources of *Legionella* are aerosolizing water systems, including outlets of the domestic water system such as faucets and shower heads. Fountains, cooling towers, spas, whirlpools, dental water lines, and humidifiers add to the list. Other sources of stagnant water can include fire sprinkler systems, eye washes, safety showers, and standing water in duct work.

Patient susceptibility is related to the immune status of the individual as well as the level of contamination of the source. Risk assessments in health care organizations traditionally focus on areas of the facility where immunocompromised individuals are housed or treated. With respect to worker safety, however, any area of the building could be problematic. Making the assumption that most health care workers are otherwise healthy, the most frequent result of infection is Pontiac Fever. Still, there will be those who have an underlying health problem that compromises their immune status and could result in Legionnaires' Disease.

Culturing

Whether to proactively culture water systems to detect the presence of *Legionella* is an ongoing debate. The CDC recommends maintaining a high index of suspicion for *Legionella* as a clinical diagnosis, but culturing only after diagnosis in hospitals that do not serve at-risk patients who require a protective environment. The CDC clearly states in its 2003 *Guidelines for Environmental Infection Control in Health Care Facilities*, "Do not conduct random, undirected, microbiologic sampling of air, water, and environmental surfaces in health care facilities."[14] *Legionella*, the agency points out, is indigenous to the water; if you culture for it, you will find it and then have to take action, even though not all occurrences will lead to disease. Likewise, OSHA advises analyzing samples only from a source suspected of being contaminated.[15]

Chapter 4: Clinically Related Risks

The CDC recommends that organizations establish a surveillance process to detect health care–associated Legionnaires Disease, including performing diagnostic laboratory tests on suspected cases, especially in at-risk patients. Whenever laboratory tests confirm a case of Legionnaires Disease or whenever two or more suspected cases occur during a six-month period, an organization should conduct an epidemiologic investigation to look for previously unidentified cases and begin intensive prospective surveillance for additional cases. An organization that treats severely immunocompromised patients should also implement culture strategies and potable water and fixture treatment measures, as outlined in the CDC's environmental infection control guidelines.[14]

Although the CDC is against routine water sampling for *Legionella*, the Maryland Department of Health and Mental Hygiene recommends that acute care hospitals in the state routinely sample plumbing systems for *Legionella*[16], and the Allegheny County (PA) Health Department says once a year is sufficient.[17] According to the Maryland guidelines, risk factors occurring at each facility, including the following, should dictate the time schedule for such assessment:

- Engineering, age, and complexity of the facility's hot water system
- Facility's remediation history and frequency
- Patient mix and the number of transplant, chemotherapy, and other immunocompromised patients served in the facility
- Prior Legionnaire's history[14]

These state health department guidelines maintain that proactively culturing the water system and treating appropriately any identified sources of *Legionella* helps maintain an environment more supportive of patient and worker safety.

The Joint Commission does not require health care organizations to routinely and proactively culture for *Legionella*. The decision is at the discretion of the organization. But, if a local authority having jurisdiction does have such a requirement, compliance with the strictest authority is always the rule of thumb.

To make an organizational decision on culturing, consult with your organization's infection control professional and make an informed decision. Some points to consider include the following:

- Surveys involving 264 hospitals in the United States, the United Kingdom, and Canada showed that nearly half of facilities found no *Legionella* in domestic water systems.
- OSHA and others have tables listing appropriate responses to various *Legionella* counts in buildings occupied by healthy people, but there are no specific guidelines available for risk zones.
- Sampling can't replace preventive maintenance or testing of patients with pneumonia.
- Any sampling should be done in conjunction with preventive/corrective measures so that constructive action is taken if contamination is found.
- Sampling can be an impetus for risk reduction and should increase communication between facility management, infection control, and the medical staff.

In any event, all sampling should follow organization policy, which should be developed in close collaboration with infection control professionals and approved by both the administration and the infection control committee.[15]

Controls

Organizations can use two main types of controls to reduce the risk of *Legionella* exposure. Organizations can use controls to reduce the risk of *Legionella* growth within a facility and/or use controls to respond to any identified infiltration of bacteria. Controls to be implemented should be documented in organization policy and procedure.

Domestic Water System

It has been previously stated that optimal temperatures for *Legionella* growth are between 80° and 120°F. The bacteria will not grow at temperatures less than 68°F and are killed above 140°F. Many health care organizations deliver hot water at the faucets or shower heads in the range of 115° to 118°F. Often, the temperature at which hot water is delivered is regulated by the state department of public health.

The AIA, in the 2001 edition of *Guidelines for Design and Construction of Hospital and Health Care Facilities*[18], recommends delivering water between 105° and 120°F. Although at the upper end of the range, these temperatures will still support *Legionella* growth. The CDC recommends delivering hot water at 124°F, but performing a scalding risk assessment for water delivered above 115°F. Furthermore, they recommend cold water storage at less than 68°F and hot water storage at greater than 140°F.[14]

If scalding is an issue, thermostatic mixing valves can be installed at the point of delivery. If these valves are used, however, the portion of the pipe between the mixing valve and the discharge of water should be self-draining to avoid any growth in that short section of pipe.

The design of the plumbing system itself is important in the control of *Legionella*. According to Kinder, "The length of piping should always be kept to a minimum, and extreme care must be exercised to avoid dead legs or dead-end piping. This is a problem that often occurs during building renovation projects when piping systems are modified leaving unused sections in place. During renovation projects, the facilities or construction manager or a designee should make periodic on-site inspections to ensure that any piping irregularities are corrected before the closing of walls and ceilings."[19]

If it is impossible to eliminate dead legs in the system, OSHA's Technical Manual suggests installing heat tracing to maintain 122°F in the lines. Frequent flushing is also recommended, along with running domestic hot water recirculation pumps continuously.

Cooling Towers

The purpose of cooling towers is to remove heat from condenser water through evaporation. The cooled water then circulates through a mechanical refrigeration unit where it absorbs heat. A fan is used to move the water through the system, thereby creating aerosolization. The typical temperature of the water in cooling towers is 85°-95°F, prime for *Legionella* growth.

Location of cooling towers is of utmost importance. They should not be located near air intakes for the building. Consideration to the prevailing winds should be given so that the cooling tower system does not draw the aerosols into the building. High efficiency drift eliminators are essential, according to OSHA, because they can reduce water loss and therefore potential personnel exposure.

Regular treatment with biocides is an important part of cooling tower maintenance. The effectiveness of chlorine and bromine has been demonstrated in controlling *Legionella* in cooling towers. Chlorine's effectiveness is greater at pH levels below 8.0, but continuous chlorination can lead to metal corrosion and wood damage in cooling towers. Bromine is less corrosive and more independent of pH. (Decorative indoor fountains should also be regularly treated with biocides to prevent *Legionella* growth.)

High concentrations of organic matter and dissolved solids in the cooling tower water will reduce the effectiveness of any biocidal agent. For this reason, each sump should be equipped with a "bleed," and make-up water should be supplied to reduce the concentration of dissolved solids.[15]

Semi-annual cleaning is a minimum for cooling towers, according to OSHA. "Normally this maintenance will be performed before initial start-up at the beginning of the cooling season and after shut-down in the fall." Additional cleaning may be required if there are high levels of biological growth. Towers that have been out of service should be cleaned and disinfected prior to being placed back online. The same is true of new towers prior to use, to eliminate any organic residue from the construction material that could contribute to *Legionella* growth.[13]

HVAC Systems

HVAC systems that are well designed and maintained should not be a source of *Legionella* in health care facilities, but they can spread contaminated aerosols. Contaminated water can come from external sources such as water drawn in through an air intake. Internal sources can include leaks into the ductwork. Humidifiers within the HVAC system can also be hazards. Four types are common:

- Heated-pan humidifiers use a heat source to evaporate water from a pan open to the air stream. Intermittent use of the device coupled with a warm pan of water may support *Legionella* growth. Contaminant-free water is essential.
- Direct stream-type humidifiers inject boiler-generated steam directly into the air stream. These systems normally operate above 158°F, and *Legionella* cannot survive at this temperature.
- Atomizing humidifiers use mechanical devices or pneumatic air to create a water mist that evaporates into the air stream. A contaminant-free water source is essential.
- Direct evaporative air coolers may be used as humidifiers. These devices mix water and air in direct contact to create a cool, wet air stream by evaporation. These devices include sumps, which may stagnate when not in use.[13]

The following methods are recommended to minimize risks in these systems:

- Minimize the use of water reservoirs, sumps, and pans
- Provide a way to drain water sumps when not in use
- Provide a "bleed" for water sumps so that dissolved solids do not form sediments
- Slope and drain sumps from the bottom so that all the water can drain out and then allow the pan to dry

- Locate HVAC fresh air intakes so that they do not draw the mist from a cooling tower, evaporative condenser, or fluid cooler into the system
- Design indirect evaporative cooling systems with the knowledge that the failure of the heat exchanger will allow wet systems to mix with the air distribution systems
- Use steam or atomizing humidifiers instead of units that use recirculated water[13]

The best course of action is to inspect, test, and maintain HVAC systems so they operate as originally designed.

Water Treatment Options

The Joint Commission expects each health care facility to have a contingency plan in place to respond to an identified *Legionella* outbreak. Included in that plan will be an investigation of the source, usually involving culturing, and subsequent treatment of the water system.

A variety of water treatment options are available. Some can be used to continuously disinfect the domestic water system, while others are best for one-time use. Many of them have both pros and cons. Following is a brief discussion of some of the water treatment options available.

Copper-Silver Ionization

The copper-silver ionization system releases copper and silver ions into the water system from electrodes in an ionization chamber. These ions bind with the *Legionella* cell membrane, killing the bacteria. This system is highly effective throughout the entire water system, including the farthest points, and it also kills the bacteria in the biofilm in the pipe. The biggest advantage to copper-silver ionization is that this system can be used continuously to prevent *Legionella* growth. If installed and used following an outbreak, this system will not only kill the bacteria, but also prevent them from growing back. Disadvantages include potential corrosion of steel or galvanized pipe, but this is not an issue with copper piping. Evidence suggests that this system works best below pH 8.5. Preventive maintenance is required, including electrode cleaning and monitoring of ion concentration. There is an initial financial investment to installing a copper-silver ionization system.

Superheating

Heating the water throughout the system to approximately 151°F will kill the *Legionella* in the system. This process requires flushing every outlet for between 5 (CDC recommendation) and 30 (PA recommendation) minutes. On the surface, this seems like a quick and inexpensive resolution, but it isn't. First, this is a very labor-intensive, highly coordinated process. Consider all the water outlets in even a small facility. Each of these must be turned on, allowed to flush, and turned off again. Proper temperatures must be determined and maintained. The elevated temperatures will probably require this process to be done during the night. What's more, as soon as the system is returned to normal temperatures, the bacteria will begin to grow again. This is at best a temporary solution.[20]

Chlorination

In this process, chlorine is injected into the water system at 10 to 50 ppm for a period of 12 to 24 hours. At these hyperchlorination levels, water may not be used. A longer-term solution uses concentrations of 1 to 2 ppm, which allows the water to be used for drinking, but at these levels, the chlorine does not attack *Legionella* in the biofilm in the pipes. At either level, chlorine can lead to leaks in the pipes. Potentially carcinogenic trihalomethanes are a byproduct of this process.[20]

Chlorine Dioxide

Chlorine dioxide is a newer treatment that has some significant advantages. It must be produced on site, and therefore requires a capital investment. It kills organisms in the biofilm, and does not produce trihalomethanes. It works in both hot and cold water between a pH range of 4 and 9. It is unclear at this point if pipes will be corroded by its use.[20]

Ultraviolet Light and Ozone

Both of these methods are point-of-use systems. Both are effective in killing *Legionella*. The problem is that these systems kill the bacteria at one point in the system, but they can grow again as they move away from the point source or in the biofilm. These systems are easy to install, but alone do not disinfect the entire system.

Different ways to manage the presence of *Legionella* in an organization's water system are available. The case study on page 102 provides an example of how one organization addressed this problem.

CASE STUDY 4-1.
Managing the Presence of *Legionella* in a Water Supply

In 2003, a trace of *Legionella* was found in the water supply at the Comprehensive Cancer Center at Johns Hopkins Hospital in Baltimore, MD. The facility, which has 154 beds and an outpatient center, successfully managed the bacteria—no cases of Legionnaire's Disease occurred.

The bacteria were found in the building's hot- and cold-water distribution systems and in the strainers where the city's potable water enters the building. The bacteria were discovered when the city's water service to the building was disrupted and heavy rains occurred due to Hurricane Isabel.

"To detect the bacteria, we used water sampling," said Greg Bova, senior operations engineer at Johns Hopkins. "Hot- and cold-water samples were taken regularly from taps throughout the building by opening the taps and letting the water flow for 30 seconds before the sample is collected. The samples were taken to our Department of Pathology lab for processing. Direct, concentrated cultures were performed from each sample."

The hospital performed active clinical surveillance on patients for *Legionella*. Any patients with symptoms of pneumonia were evaluated for Legionnaire's Disease with a urinary antigen test. Testing was not conducted on staff, but employees concerned about their own health—possibly because they were immunocompromised—were told to consult their personal physicians.

"Water restrictions were immediately imposed for the entire building," Bova added. "We placed prohibitions on showers, tub bathing, drinking from water fountains, using ice, and drinking water from ice machines. Bottled water and waterless hand cleaner were provided, ice was provided from other buildings, and sponge baths were offered."

To remove the bacteria, hot- and cold-water systems were flushed and treated with elevated levels of chlorine dioxide disinfectant for six hours. Chlorine dioxide was pumped into water mains to maintain elevated, detectable levels at all fixtures.

Bova gave several reasons why Johns Hopkins chose to use chlorine dioxide instead of superheating water or using chlorine: "Superheating can't be done on cold-water systems because hot-water temperatures over 160°F are required to kill the bacteria. Superheating has limited effect on fixtures because of the anti-scald devices that prevent hot water from exceeding 115°F at the fixtures. Superheating also has a limited effect on biofilm in the piping and minimal residual effect.

"Chlorine treatment requires pumping high levels of chlorine into the hot- and cold-water piping and at all fixtures. Once the chlorine is in the piping system, sinks, showers, and toilets, they can't be used for 3 to 24 hours depending on the level of chlorine used. When they are ready to use, the water system must be purged until the levels of chlorine are below EPA maximum limits."

Using chlorine has other disadvantages. The water restrictions and flushing of highly chlorinated water and the strong odors that come with high levels of chlorine can be disruptive to patients, visitors, and staff in the building. Also, elevated levels of chlorine are corrosive to the piping system and chlorine has minimal residual effect on biofilm and bacteria even when used continuously at the maximum levels allowed by the EPA.

Chlorine dioxide, however, is EPA-approved for potable water disinfection and it is documented to be over five times more effective at killing bacteria than chlorine, Bova said. "During remediation treatments with chlorine dioxide, drinking is prohibited but flushing toilets and washing hands at sinks are allowed. Chlorine dioxide odors are not noticeable during treatments; it has an excellent impact on biofilm and bacteria; and it has significant residual effect," Bova explained.

If *Legionella* bacteria are detected in water systems at levels requiring corrective action, the organization should consider implementing an awareness program to inform patients, visitors, and employees of the biological hazard.

For health care facilities, management of waterborne bacteria, not prevention, is the right approach. "These events are not always preventable, but their impact can be minimized and made manageable," Bova advised. "Closing of water valves, flushing the piping systems, and cleaning water devices such as aerators and strainers will limit the bacterial loading of the distribution system. If necessary, self-imposed water restrictions may be applied until flushing and treatment of the water system can be done. It's important to review your *Legionella* control and prevention procedures and develop surveillance programs, water-treatment programs, and remediation plans."[21]

Training

Typically, health care organizations do not conduct routine training programs about *Legionella*. At its worst, it is an infrequent issue, and more likely has adverse patient effects than impacts on worker safety. In the event of an outbreak, however, the Joint Commission, OSHA, and the CDC would expect an employee awareness program to tell employees about the potential outbreak and provide information about the disease and its symptoms to alleviate fears and promote early recognition. In addition, the facility would be required to take the appropriate steps necessary to ensure that the workplace provides safe and healthful working conditions.

On recognition of more than one case of Legionellosis in the work place, the following should be provided:

- An employee training session that provides basic information about the disease, information known about the source of the cases, and actions being taken to investigate the problem
- An ongoing general information service to provide updates and answer questions that may arise among employees
- Medical and psychological counseling services when an outbreak has occurred

The OSHA Technical Manual provides some frequently asked questions to assist employers in providing this information.[13]

ETHYLENE OXIDE, FORMALDEHYDE, AND GLUTARALDEHYDE

The three chemicals discussed in this section have some things in common, as well as some differences. All three have common but specific uses in health care organizations, and can be highly hazardous when inappropriately used or as the source of an accidental exposure.

Fortunately, less hazardous substances have been identified as possible substitutes for these chemicals. And at least for ethylene oxide (ETO) and glutaraldehyde, both used as sterilants, the substitutes are gaining popularity and many organizations are making the switch. Formaldehyde, (frequently used as 10% formalin solution) is a tissue fixative, and remains in common use in clinical laboratories, particularly in the histology section. Because the fixative can make a difference in the ultimate appearance of the tissue used for pathological diagnosis, most institutions are reluctant to adopt a less-hazardous alternative.

Standards and Regulations

The Joint Commission addresses ETO, formaldehyde, and glutaraldehyde in EC.3.10, which deals with hazardous materials and waste. Many of the EPs associated with this standard discuss important issues surrounding the safe use of ETO, formaldehyde, and glutaraldehyde. For example, EP3 addresses the processes that an organization must undertake to manage hazardous chemicals from "cradle to grave"; that is, selecting, handling, storing, transporting, using, and disposing them from receipt through final disposal. Other EPs discuss the creation and maintenance of a hazardous materials inventory (EP2), adequate and appropriate space and equipment for handling and storage (EP7), and emergency procedures for spills and exposures (EP9). Of course, the overall requirement for a safe and effective environmental health and safety program found in EC.1.10 also applies, as do the training requirements in HR.2.10, HR.2.20, and HR.2.30.

STANDARDS *Joint Commission Standards that Implicitly Address Ethylene Oxide, Formaldehyde, and Glutaraldehyde*

➤ EC.1.10, Safety Management; EC.1.20, Environmental Tours; EC.3.10, Hazardous Materials & Waste Management (EP1, EP2, EP7, EP8, EP9, EP10, EP12, EP13); EC.9.10, Monitoring Environmental Conditions; EC.9.20, Analyzing Environmental Issues; EC.9.30, Improving the Environment
➤ HR.2.10, Initial Job Training; HR.2.20, Roles & Responsibilities; HR.2.30, Ongoing Education

Although OSHA has specific regulations addressing ETO and formaldehyde, no comprehensive OSHA regulation exists for glutaraldehyde. Any evidence that employees were exposed to glutaraldehyde levels with the potential for physical harm would be cited under OSHA's general duty clause[22] or other OSHA standards (for example, 29CFR 1910.1020, Access to Employee Exposure and Medical Records). The ethylene oxide standard is found at 29CFR 1910.1047,[†] and 29CFR 1910.1048 is OSHA's formaldehyde standard.[‡] Although the Joint Commission does not take an active role in facilities' compliance with these standards, OSHA does require compliance. The following section discusses OSHA's requirements in general. Specific information about the requirements can be obtained at OSHA's Web site, http://www.osha.gov.

Hazard

Ethylene Oxide

ETO is a flammable and colorless gas. It is typically used in sterile processing departments to sterilize surgical instruments. At toxic levels, it smells like ether. Exposure to ETO in hospital settings is usually through inhalation. Symptoms of acute exposure include eye pain, sore throat, blurred vision, and difficulty breathing. Additional effects are dizziness, nausea, headache, convulsions, and blisters. Vomiting and coughing can result, along with drowsiness, weakness, and lack of coordination. Nerve damage, peripheral paralysis, muscle weakness, and impaired thinking and memory have also been associated with exposure.[24, 25] In addition, "clinical evidence of adverse effects associated with the exposure to ETO is present in the form of increased incidence of cancer in laboratory animals (leukemia, stomach, brain), mutation in offspring in animals, and resorptions and spontaneous abortions in animals and human populations respectively. Findings in humans and experimental animals exposed to airborne concentrations of ETO also indicate damage to the genetic material (DNA)."[25]

Formaldehyde

Formaldehyde is a strong-smelling, colorless gas. Most often it is present in mixtures with alcohol and water, called "formalin," which is 37%-50% formaldehyde and 6%-15% alcohol stabilizer. As with ETO, healthcare exposure to formaldehyde is primarily via inhalation. Symptoms of acute exposure to either liquid or vapor include eye and respiratory irritation. Exposure can cause symptoms of bronchial asthma. Tolerance to low levels of exposure can develop within 1-2 hours, thus permitting the worker to remain in the environment even while the risk increases. Skin contact can cause irritation and contact dermatitis at low levels.[26] Chronic exposure to formaldehyde vapors can cause laryngitis, bronchitis or bronchial pneumonia, or conjunctivitis. Animal studies have linked nasal tumors to formaldehyde exposure.[27] Studies also show an increased risk of cancer of the nose and sinuses, nasopharyngeal and oropharyngeal cancer, and lung cancer in humans. Smoking may contribute to the effects of formaldehyde exposure.[26]

Glutaraldehyde

Glutaraldehyde is a component of cold sterilants sold under a variety of brand names. It is used to sterilize instruments that are heat-sensitive, such as respiratory therapy equipment, bronchoscopes, physical therapy whirlpools, and so forth.[28] Liquid or vapor exposure to glutaraldehyde can cause severe eye irritation. Higher concentrations can burn the skin. Inhalation causes irritation to the nose, throat, and respiratory tract, resulting in cough, wheezing, nausea, headaches, nosebleeds, and dizziness. Some workers are very sensitive to glutaraldehyde and can have strong reactions to low-level exposures, such as sudden asthma attacks. Longer-term exposures can cause skin allergy and/or chronic eczema.[28]

---

† It is found in subpart Z of the OSHA regulation, addressing "toxic and hazardous substances." Four non-mandatory appendices are associated with this standard:
- Appendix A   Substance Safety Data Sheet for Ethylene Oxide
- Appendix B   Substance Technical Guidelines for Ethylene Oxide
- Appendix C   Medical Surveillance Guidelines for Ethylene Oxide
- Appendix D   Sampling and Analytical Methods for Ethylene Oxide

Much of the appendix material is an expansion of topics addressed in the standard itself. Although non-mandatory, appendix A contains an entire section on "Sterilant Use of ETO in Hospitals and Healthcare Facilities," which provides additional guidance in workplace design and practices.

There is an exception to the applicability of this standard, "where objective data are reasonably relied upon that demonstrate that the product is not capable of releasing ETO in airborne concentrations at or above the action level under the expected conditions of processing, use, or handling that will cause the greatest possible release." This exception will probably not apply to most health care settings.

‡ This requirement has four associated appendices:
- Appendix A   Substance Technical Guidelines for Formalin
- Appendix B   Sampling Strategy and Analytical Methods for Formaldehyde
- Appendix C   Medical Surveillance – Formaldehyde
- Appendix D   Medical Disease Questionnaire

An appendix E on qualitative and quantitative fit testing procedures has been removed. Like the ETO standard, much of the appendix material expands upon topics covered in the standard itself. But unlike ETO, only appendix D, the medical disease questionnaire is non-mandatory.

Figure 4-3. Exposure Limits[24, 30]

	ETHYLENE OXIDE	FORMALDEHYDE
Permissible Exposure Limit (PEL) (8 hr. TWA)	1 ppm	0.75 ppm
Short Term Exposure Limit (STEL) (15 min. sampling)	5 ppm	2 ppm
Action Level (8 hr. TWA)	0.5 ppm	0.5 ppm

Worker exposure to these toxins must not exceed the limits set by OSHA.

Source: U.S. Department of Labor, Occupational Safety and Health Administration.

Exposure

Facilities that use formaldehyde or ETO must monitor their workers to determine worker exposures to these agents. Other requirements are also in place when workers are exposed to an amount that reaches the action level or the short-term exposure limit (STEL).§ Limits for ETO and formaldehyde exposure are shown in Figure 4-3.

Because OSHA has no comprehensive standard for glutaraldehyde there is no specific PEL; however, the American College of Governmental Industrial Hygienists (ACGIH) has established a ceiling level threshold limit value (TLV) of 0.2 ppm, above which employees cannot be exposed.[22]

To determine exposure levels, organizations should monitor employees for exposure. A process of representative sampling may be used as long as it accurately determines the concentrations of the chemicals to which employees may be exposed and does not underestimate the exposure of any employee. Initial monitoring must be undertaken, and repeated with any change in the process, equipment, or control measures.

The frequency of monitoring depends on the employee exposure level. For ETO or formaldehyde, if employee exposure is above the action level, but at or below the time weighted average (TWA), OSHA requires monitoring to be repeated for that employee at least every six months. If exposure is above the 8 hour TWA for ETO, monitoring must be repeated for that employee at least every three months. For formaldehyde, employee exposure at or above STEL must be repeated annually under worst-case conditions.[23, 29] If any employee reports symptoms of exposure, the employee must be provided with a medical evaluation and his or her exposure must be monitored.

Because OSHA does not have a comprehensive standard for glutaraldehyde, there is no OSHA-mandated requirement for monitoring employee exposure. It is, however, considered good practice to perform baseline exposure monitoring to determine exposure. If this level is below the 0.2 ppm ACGIH ceiling limit, it is not necessary to perform ongoing monitoring unless something changes in the process. Employees must be notified of their monitoring results within 15 days, either in person or by posted notice, and have the opportunity to observe any monitoring of employee exposure.

It is important to maintain monitoring records for each employee. According to OSHA some of the information housed in such records must include the date of measurement; operation being monitored; sampling and analysis methods; the number, duration, time, and results of samples; and the names, job classifications, social security numbers, and exposures of the monitored employees. Exposure monitoring records must be kept for 30 years. Where the concentration of ETO, formaldehyde, or glutaraldehyde is above safe limits, the areas should be regulated with access limited to authorized persons. These areas are to be labeled to keep out unauthorized employees. OSHA requires specific language for signage. This language is available at http://www.osha.gov.

Controls

Engineering and work practice controls should be used to maintain the lowest possible exposure levels for ETO, formaldehyde, and glutaraldehyde. For formaldehyde, engineering controls could include

---

§ OSHA has an exception for formaldehyde, "Where the employer documents, using objective data, that the presence of formaldehyde or formaldehyde-releasing products in the workplace cannot result in airborne concentrations of formaldehyde that would cause any employee to be exposed at or above the action level or the STEL under foreseeable conditions of use, the employer will not be required to measure employee exposure to formaldehyde."[33]

local exhaust ventilation. For example, in an area where the pathologists section the surgical specimens that have been fixed in formalin, exhaust units placed at the level of and immediately adjacent to the cutting table remove the vapors, preventing exposure.

To limit exposure to glutaraldehyde, it is advisable to use glutaraldehydein rooms that are well-ventilated and large enough to ensure adequate dilution of the vapor; 10 air changes per hour is the minimum. Glutaraldehyde should not be used in exam rooms, where patient exposure may result. A fume hood provides local exhaust ventilation for glutaraldehyde use. Capture velocity of at least 100 feet per minute is recommended. Glutaraldehyde should be stored in closed containers.[28]

The OSHA standard for ETO states that engineering and work practice controls may not be feasible in all situations. "Engineering controls are generally infeasible for the following operations: collection of quality assurance sampling from sterilized materials, removal of biological indicators from sterilized materials. . . changing of ethylene oxide tanks on sterilizers. . ."[23] Under these circumstances, or where engineering and work practice controls are ineffective at reducing exposure, respiratory protection must be made available to employees. In both cases, a respiratory protection program must be in place, as discussed in Chapter Three.

Respirator selection for ETO, formaldehyde, and glutaraldehyde is dependent on the anticipated level of exposure. A full facepiece respirator with substance-approved cartridges or canisters provides the minimum protection. In emergency situations, when the exposure level is unknown, SCBA (self-contained breathing apparatus) with positive pressure full facepiece or combination supplied-air full facepiece positive pressure respirator with an auxiliary self-contained air supply must be used.[23,29]

Other PPE, such as a face and eye protection, is required if splashing formaldehyde or glutaraldehyde is a danger. In this case, eyewash facilities should be available in the immediate work area.

Glove material for full protection from glutaraldehyde includes butyl rubber, nitrile, and Viton®. For exposures of shorter duration, polyethylene gloves may be used. Latex gloves will provide protection only for short-term incidental contact.[28]

Medical Surveillance

OSHA requires medical surveillance to be made available to employees who are exposed to ETO or formaldehyde above the action level, STEL, in an emergency situation, or when they develop symptoms of exposure. Although not required by a specific OSHA standard, it may also be prudent for organizations to provide medical surveillance for glutaraldehyde exposure above the TLV.

OSHA requires that a medical examination must be made available prior to assignment to an area of elevated exposure and at least annually thereafter. In the case of ETO, a medical and work history must be taken that addresses symptoms related to the pulmonary, hematologic, neurologic, and reproductive systems, in addition to the eyes and skin. For formaldehyde, OSHA provides a medical disease questionnaire that is designed to obtain the relevant work history.

The OSHA physician performing the examination must be provided with the relevant OSHA standards, a description of the employee's job duties related to exposure, the representative exposure level, a description of PPE and respiratory protection used, and information from previous medical examinations (under the employer's control).[23,29] For formaldehyde exposure based on an emergency, the physician must also have a description of how the emergency occurred and the potential exposure. The physician must provide a written opinion regarding whether the employee has any medical condition that would place him or her at an increased risk of material impairment of health from exposure. The written opinion must include any recommendations for exposure limitations or changes in the use of PPE. The opinion must include a statement that the employee has been informed of the outcome of the examination, and the employee must receive a written report within 15 days of the examination.

Records of all medical surveillance related to ETO, formaldehyde, and glutaraldehyde must be maintained. OSHA's Access to Employee Exposure and Medical Records standard requires all other work-related medical records to be maintained. (See 29CFR 1910.1020 at http://www.osha.gov.) OSHA-specific standards for ETO and formaldehyde require that records include the employee's name and social security number, the physician's written opinion, any employee medical complaints related to exposure, and medical examination results, including health history or questionnaire. These records must be kept for 30 years.

Training

To ensure worker safety, organizations should train employees on the hazards associated with ETO, formaldehyde, and glutaraldehyde where appropriate. Employees should be trained on initial assignment and at least annually thereafter. OSHA has specific

requirements regarding the content of such training programs. Following is a list of those requirements.
- The ETO program must include:
- The requirements of the OSHA standard
- Any operations involving the presence of ETO
- The medical surveillance program
- Ways to detect the presence or release of ETO
- The physical and health hazards of exposure to ETO
- Protective measures, such as work practices, emergency procedures, and PPE
- The hazard communication program

Formaldehyde training requirements are as follows:
- The requirements of the OSHA standard and the contents of the MSDS
- The medical surveillance program
- Instructions to immediately report adverse signs and symptoms
- Operations where formaldehyde is present
- Safe work practices
- Purpose, use, and limitations of PPE
- Spills, emergencies, and clean up procedures
- Engineering and work practice controls
- Emergency procedures

Again, with no specific OSHA standard, there is no standard-specified training for employees with glutaraldehyde exposure. However, under the Hazard Communication Program (see Chapter One), all employees must be instructed about the chemicals to which they are exposed.

HAZARDOUS DRUGS, REPRODUCTIVE HAZARDS, AND ANESTHETIC GAS

The three topics for this section have very blurred boundaries. Hazardous drugs frequently pose reproductive hazards and include anesthetic gas, which also has potential reproductive ramifications. Accordingly, these topics will all be discussed together in this section.

Of course, exposure to some of these drugs pose other potential hazards. Several of these hazards will also be highlighted in this section.

Standards and Regulations

In addition to the general requirement for an effective environmental health and safety program in EC.1.10, the risks associated with hazardous drugs, reproductive hazards, and anesthetic gas more specifically fall under the requirements of EC.3.10, hazardous materials and waste.

Applicable requirements are interspersed throughout the latter standard. For example, EP4 calls for management of the cradle-to-grave processes for chemotherapeutic materials and EP5 for radioactive materials, both of which can fall into the reproductive hazard category. Of course, chemotherapeutic materials are also hazardous drugs.

STANDARDS *Joint Commission Standards Implicitly Addressing Hazardous Drugs, Reproductive Hazards, and Anesthetic Gas*

➤ EC.1.10, Safety Management; EC.3.10, Hazardous Materials & Waste Management (EP4, EP5)

OSHA does not have a comprehensive regulation that specifically addresses hazardous drugs. However, OSHA does provide guidance on these topics. For example, the Standards for General Industry, specifically the Hazard Communication Standard, discuss hazardous drugs and training requirements. Any employee medical records related to workplace exposure are covered under OSHA's Access to Employee Exposure and Medical Records standard. Gloves and other PPE used for protection are covered under the Personal Protective Equipment standards. The OSHA Technical Manual also discusses occupational exposure to hazardous drugs. The OSHA Web site, http://www.osha.gov, contains a "Safety and Health Topics" page for reproductive hazards. Standards addressing these hazards are specific to chemicals, such as ethylene oxide, which was discussed previously.

HAZARDS

Hazardous Drugs
OSHA's Technical Manual describes hazardous drugs as those that "may pose occupational risk to employees through acute and chronic workplace exposure."[31]

Four characteristics are considered for classifying a drug as hazardous, including genotoxicity, carcinogenicity, teratogenicity or fertility impairment, and serious organ or other toxic manifestation at low doses in experimental animals or treated patients.[31]

Figure 4-4. Hazardous Drugs[31]

Altretamine	Dacarbazine	Interferon-A	Plicamycin
Aminoglutethimide	Dactinomycin	Isotretinoin	Procarbazine
Azathioprine	Daunorubucin	Leuprolide	Ribavirin
L-Asparaginase	Diethylstilbestrol	Levamisole	Streptozocin
Bleomycin	Doxorubicin	Lomustine	Tamoxifen
Busulfan	Estradiol	Mechlorethamine	Testolactone
Carboplatin	Estramustine	Medroxyprogesterone	Thioguanine
Carmustine	Ethinyl Estradiol	Megestrol	Thiotepa
Chlorambucil	Etoposide	Melphalan	Uracil Mustard
Chloramphenicol	Floxuridine	Mercaptopurine	Vidarabine
Chlorotianisene	Fluorouracil	Methotrexate	Vinblastine
Chlorozotocin	Flutamide	Mitomycin	Vincristine
Cyclosporin	Ganciclovir	Mitotane	Zidvudine
Cisplatin	Hydroxyurea	Mitoxantrone	
Cyclophosphamide	Idarubicin	Nafarelin	
Cytarrabine	Ifosfamide	Pipobroman	

These are only some of the drugs which can be hazardous to health care workers.
Source: U.S. Department of Labor, Occupational Safety and Health Administration.

Figure 4-4 contains a listing of some hazardous drugs. This list was derived from those of several facilities and other sources at the time the OSHA Technical Manual was prepared. This is not an exhaustive list, nor is there complete industry consensus on the list. Investigational drugs are not included, but they are prudently handled as hazardous drugs until enough information regarding their safety is available to exclude them.

Organizations would be wise to seek professional judgment by qualified pharmacology and/or toxicology personnel in designating hazardous drugs for an individual organization. Essentially, this becomes a risk assessment process, as required by Joint Commission standard EC.1.10, EP4.

Unlike chemicals, which frequently have designated exposure limits, the effects of hazardous drugs are dependent on the degree of absorption and its biological impact, which have individual variables. Typically, drugs are demonstrated to be toxic based on three factors:
- Action Mechanism: Binding directly to genetic material or impact on protein synthesis at the cellular level
- Animal Data: Demonstrating carcinogenic, mutagenic, and teratogenic effects
- Human Data: At therapeutic levels, demonstrated carcinogenicity, contribution to chromosomal aberrations, reproductive dysfunction, and impact on other organ systems[31]

The above characteristics are essentially true of chemotherapeutic agents, which may not differentiate between malignant and nonmalignant cells. It is recommended that all animal carcinogens also be treated as human carcinogens.

Exposure may come not only from the preparation, administration, or spills of these drugs, but also from caring for patients who have received them. High concentrations of some chemotherapeutic materials may be present in the excreta of the patients, hence urine or soiled linen may be another route of exposure.

Disposing of materials contaminated with these drugs, such as vials, gloves, gowns, linen, and so forth, may expose environmental services staff.

Reproductive Hazards

Radiation, many chemicals, and certain drugs can all pose risks for reproductive issues. Figure 4-5 provides a list of reproductive hazards specific to female health

Figure 4-5. Chemical and Physical Female Reproductive Hazards[32]

AGENT	OBSERVED EFFECTS	POTENTIALLY EXPOSED WORKERS
Cancer Treatment Drugs	Infertility, birth defects, low birth weight	Health care workers, including nurses, housekeepers, pharmacists
Ionizing Radiation (x-rays and gamma rays)	Infertility, miscarriage, birth defects, low birth weight, developmental disorders, childhood cancers	Health care workers, dental personnel, atomic workers

Certain hazardous treatments pose a threat specifically for female health care workers.
Source: U.S. Department of Public Health, Centers for Disease Control and Prevention.

---

care workers, as provided by the National Institute for Occupational Safety and Health (NIOSH), which is part of the CDC.

In addition to the previously mentioned hazards, a number of infectious diseases to which female health care workers can be exposed may also pose a reproductive risk. These include cytomegalovirus (CMV), hepatitis B virus (see discussion on Bloodborne Pathogens in this chapter), Human Immunodeficiency Virus (HIV) (see BBP section), Human Parvovirus B19, rubella (German measles), toxoplasmosis, and varicella-zoster virus (chicken pox).[32]

The companion NIOSH publication on male reproductive health lists primarily chemicals—many of which are not in common use in health care—as potential male reproductive hazards. However, the following exposures and their potential effects may apply:

- Radiation: Lowered number of sperm, abnormal sperm shape, altered sperm transfer, altered hormones/sexual performance
- Heat: Lowered number of sperm, altered sperm transfer
- Welding: Abnormal sperm shape, altered sperm transfer
- Mercury vapor: Altered hormones/sexual performance[33]

In both males and females, the length of exposure and the hazard have an influence on the impact. In addition personal factors come into consideration, and not all who are exposed will experience adverse effects.

Anesthetic Gases

Anesthetic gas exposure typically occurs from waste anesthetic gas (WAG) escaping into the operating room environment. This can occur due to leaks from various components of the anesthesia delivery system, improper practices, spillage, poorly fitting face masks, or improperly inflated airway cuffs. The latter two exposures are then directly attributable to the patient's breath. In the post-anesthesia care unit (PACU, or recovery room), the exposure is exclusively from the patients' respiration and therefore staff can be exposed to multiple gases.

Two types of anesthesia are of concern: nitrous oxide, which is a gas, and the vapors of halogenated agents, which include halothane, enflurane, isoflurane, desflurane, and sevoflurane.

OSHA has not established permissible exposure limits for these anesthetics. NIOSH has issued a recommended exposure limit (REL) for nitrous oxide of 25 ppm as a TWA during the period of anesthetic administration. The NIOSH ceiling level for halogenated agents is a concentration of 2 ppm over a one-hour time period. There are no RELs for isoflurane, desflurane, and sevoflurane. ACGIH has issued TLV-TWAs (during an eight-hour workday) as follows:

- Nitrous Oxide: 50 ppm
- Halothane: 50 ppm
- Enflurane: 75 ppm

Animal studies of the health effects of nitrous oxide have shown reproductive and developmental abnormalities with exposure to high concentrations. In addition, a human study involving female dental assistants exposed to unscavenged nitrous oxide for five or more hours per week demonstrated reduced fertility. Other human studies have indicated an increased risk of spontaneous abortion from nitrous oxide exposure.[34] Nitrous oxide has also been linked to neurologic, renal, and liver disease, as well as decreased mental performance, audiovisual ability, and manual dexterity.[35]

Halogenated agents were investigated in both human and animal studies and have been shown to cause reproductive problems such as spontaneous abortions and congenital abnormality. Furthermore, these outcomes have also been seen in wives of exposed male health care workers.[34]

Controls

As with other hazards, the effective controls for hazardous drugs, waste anesthetic gases, and other reproductive hazards involve engineering controls (for example, waste anesthetic gas scavenging systems, biological safety cabinets for hazardous drug preparation), administrative, and work practice controls PPE. Common sense practices to avoid chemical exposure include storing chemicals in sealed containers; washing hands after use or any hand contact; before eating, drinking, or smoking; and using PPE to avoid skin contact.

Hazardous Drugs

Although not required, development of a hazardous drug safety and health plan is a recommended administrative and work practice control to both protect employees and keep exposures at the lowest possible level. The plan could also serve as a comprehensive source for including required elements such as PPE, hazard communication, and medical record maintenance.

ASHP recommends the following plan inclusions:
- Standard operating procedures for exposed employees
- Employer criteria to determine and implement controls
- Functioning ventilation and other equipment
- Employee information and training
- Circumstances for approval and use of FDA investigational drugs
- Medical examinations for exposed personnel
- Designating personnel responsible for the plan

Other plan inclusions may include procedures for safe waste removal and decontamination procedures, if applicable. After the plan is created it should be reviewed at least annually and updated as necessary.[31]

As part of the above-mentioned plan, organizations should consider establishing a designated hazardous drug handling area and/or creating a designated hazardous drug preparation area.

A recommended engineering control to address hazardous drugs is class II or III biological safety cabinets (BSC). If these are not available, it is advisable to send the patient to a facility where they are used. Class II BSCs have downward airflow and HEPA filters, but there are differences regarding the amount of recirculated air within the cabinet, whether the air is vented to the room or outside, and whether the ducts are under positive or negative pressure. Those venting to the outside and without air recirculation offer the most protection. Class III BSCs are totally enclosed and under negative pressure, with all air HEPA filtered. These cabinets may be thought of as "glove boxes," with all work done through attached gloves. Administration of aerosolized drugs, such as ribavirin and pentamidine, must be done using engineering controls; for example, a treatment booth with local exhaust ventilation, or isolation rooms with separate HEPA-filtered ventilation.

PPE controls for hazardous drugs include gloves and gowns. Eye and face protection should also be used for hazardous drug preparation, and when biological safety cabinets are not yet available, respiratory protection provides a last line of defense for inhalational exposure. For administering hazardous drugs, the gloves, gowns, and chemical eye protection should be used.

For home care delivery of hazardous drugs, the same PPE should be available, but in addition, emergency procedures, including emergency contact information, and spill kits should be available.

All glove materials that have been tested allow some permeability to hazardous drugs, although some thicker latex gloves seem to perform best with certain drugs. The glove thickness is the most important protection; therefore, double gloving is recommended. Gloves should be changed at least hourly, or as soon as they are torn, punctured, or contaminated with a spill.

Gowns should have a closed front, long sleeves, and elastic or knit closed cuffs. A low-permeability fabric is best. The least permeable fabrics are laminated or polyethylene coated. A gown made completely of these fabrics is not necessary; having the fabrics on the front and sleeves of the gown is acceptable and more comfortable to wear. To prevent exposure at the cuff, the cuff should be tucked under the glove. If double gloves are used, the inner glove should go under the gown's cuff and the outer glove should go over the cuff.

According to the OSHA Technical Manual, if a BSC is not available for hazardous drug preparation, a NIOSH-approved respirator for hazardous drug preparation must be worn. A powered, air purifying respirator (PAPR) is recommended, but this should not be a substitute for the BSC engineering control.

Chemical barrier eye and face protection should be worn whenever there is a risk of splashes or aerosols. Eyewash facilities should be available in the work area.

All disposables involved in hazardous drug preparation, including gowns and gloves, should be disposed of as hazardous drug waste. Covered sharps disposal containers should be available within the BSC. All work within the BSC should be done on a disposable, plastic-backed paper liner, which is changed as needed or at least after every shift. A covered disposable container should be available for excess liquid.

Disposal of waste contaminated with hazardous drugs should be in thick, leak-proof plastic bags that are distinctively color-coded. Bags containing hazardous chemicals should be labeled according to the requirements of the Hazard Communication Standard (see Chapter One). Other bags of hazardous drug waste should be labeled as such. Disposal should be in accordance with applicable EPA, state, and local regulations.

Spills of hazardous drugs should be cleaned up immediately by appropriately trained personnel. Small spills are defined by American Society of Health-System Pharmacists (ASHP) as being less than 5 ml, large spills are greater than 5 ml. Small spills should be cleaned wearing appropriate PPE, including gowns, appropriate double gloves, and goggles. Respiratory protection should be used for powder or liquid spills where either an aerosol or airborne powder is present. OSHA recommends that spills should be cleaned up as follows:
- "Liquids should be wiped with absorbent gauze pads; solids should be wiped with wet absorbent gauze. The spill areas should then be cleaned three times using a detergent solution followed by clean water."
- "Any broken glass fragments should be picked up using a small scoop (never the hands) and placed in a sharps container. The container should then go into a hazardous drug disposal bag, along with used absorbent pads and any other contaminated waste."[31]

Areas where large spills occur should be isolated and cleaned by specially trained personnel. Liquids should be "gently covered with absorbent sheets or spill-control pads or pillows. If a powder is involved, damp cloths or towels should be used."[31]

Organizations should create a hazardous drug spill kit. Contents for this kit could include chemical splash goggles, pairs of gloves, utility gloves, a low-permeability gown, sheets of absorbent material, spill-control pillows, a sharps container, a small scoop, and large hazardous drug waste disposal bags.[31]

Anesthetic Gas
All anesthesia machines are subject to leakage. Leaks can be due to loose fittings; defective gaskets; worn, missing, or defective parts; and so forth. Leaks can also be due to a mask that does not properly fit the patient, or any other potentially open portion of the system. Obviously, the anesthesia machine should be thoroughly checked before use to minimize the leaks.

A WAG scavenging system is an engineering control to collect gas and vapors at the point of overflow. A WAG ventilation system is an engineering control that can remove gas and vapors from the room. These systems are included in most new equipment. A scavenging system has the following components:
- Gas collection assembly: Collects excess gas at the site of emission and delivers it to transfer tubing.
- Transfer tubing: Conveys gas to the interface.
- Interface: Provides positive (and sometimes negative) pressure relief to protect the patient's lungs from the pressure of the scavenging system.
- Gas disposal assembly tubing: Conducts gas from the interface to the gas disposal assembly.
- Gas disposal assembly: Conveys excess gas to a point where it can be safely discharged into the atmosphere.[34]

General dilution ventilation can be combined with a gas scavenging system to reduce staff exposure to waste anesthetic gas. Ceiling supply registers direct the air downward, with exhaust registers located near the floor level.

Good work practices can also aid in minimizing exposure to WAG. Many of these are specific to the clinical staff in the operating room, such as appropriately fitting the face mask, positioning the tracheal tube, and extubation. Clinical engineering and facilities staff also participate in some work practice controls, including monitoring WAG concentration, identifying and correcting sources of leakage, determining adequacy and proper functioning of the scavenging system, and ensuring the provision of appropriate air exchanges.

As mentioned previously, nitrous oxide is a type of anesthetic gas that is of concern regarding exposure issues. NIOSH recommends the following to reduce exposure to nitrous oxide:
- Leak test equipment
- Monitoring air in the worker's personal breathing zone
- Monitoring the room air
- Preventing leakage from the anesthetic delivery system through proper maintenance and inspection
- Eliminating or replacing any loose fitting connections, loosely assembled or deformed slip joints and threaded connections, and defective or worn seals, gaskets, breathing bags, and hoses
- Securely fitting masks
- Sufficient flow rates (45 liters per minute) for the exhaust system
- Properly vented vacuum pumps[35]

Administrative controls that can be used to reduce exposure to waste anesthetic gas include a program of routine and regular maintenance, a WAG monitoring program, an orientation program for staff, medical surveillance, and compliance with applicable laws and regulations.

PPE controls can also be used to reduce exposure; however, they should not be substituted for higher level controls. In fact, traditional PPE, such as gowns and gloves, will add nothing to the protection against exposure to waste anesthetic gas, nor will HEPA filtration. Air-supplied respirators would eliminate the exposure, but are not comfortable for all-day wear or practical in an OR setting. Therefore, the engineering controls described above are essential.

Cleaning up spills does call for PPE, including gloves, eye and face protection, and chemical protective clothing. Neoprene and nitrile are the best materials for gloves and body protection. Respirators should be used as appropriate. For a large spill, the minimum protection is a type "C" supplied-air respirator with a full facepiece, helmet, or hood. This should be operated in continuous-flow mode.[34]

Medical Surveillance

Hazardous Drugs
OSHA's Technical Manual[31] recommends preplacement medical examinations for employees who will be exposed to chemical hazards. Annual re-examinations are suggested, but recommended at least every two to three years. The employee should also be examined in the case of accidental acute exposure and upon job termination. The physician should be provided with information about the employee's job duties, potential levels of exposure, and a description of PPE used. The exam should include a complete occupational history that includes the drugs handled, the length of exposure on a weekly basis, and the number of preparations or administrations per week. Records of the exam must be kept for the duration of employment plus 30 years. The focus of the examination should be the skin, mucous membranes, cardiopulmonary and lymphatic systems, and the liver. The reproductive status of the employee should be considered, with a discussion of relevant issues.

Anesthetic Gas
The OSHA recommendations for medical surveillance of employees exposed to anesthetic gas include preplacement and annual review. The preplacement review is to establish a baseline and the annual update is primarily for educational purposes. A final review should be conducted at the time of employment termination. These reviews may be accomplished via medical questionnaires, with examinations offered to employees based on their responses. The questionnaire should record a detailed work history, including past exposure to WAG, and a medical history emphasizing hepatic, renal, neurological, cardiovascular, and reproductive functions.

Employees should be advised of the need to report any health problems that may be related to their exposure, and of potential risks of exposure, including spontaneous abortions, congenital abnormalities in children, and the effects on the liver and kidneys. The OSHA Access to Employee Exposure and Medical Records standard requires that all work-related medical records, including records of medical surveillance and any abnormal pregnancy outcomes of employees exposed to WAG, must be kept for the duration of employment plus 30 years.[34]

Training
As with all other types of hazards, the Joint Commission recommends and the OSHA Hazard Communication Standard requires that organizations educate their employees about the risks involved with workplace exposure to chemicals, including hazardous drugs, anesthetic gases, and other reproductive hazards. Staff should be trained on how to properly handle these items and how to identify potential exposure issues.

CONCLUSION
Because of the nature of health care, workers in health care facilities can be exposed to dangerous infectious agents, chemicals, and gases that can impact their health and safety. Organizations that take a proactive approach to identifying risks and implementing controls to minimize those risks can further protect the employees and the patients entrusted to their care. ■

Chapter 4: Clinically Related Risks

References

1. U.S. Department of Labor: Occupational Safety and Health Administration: *Bloodborne Pathogens.* http://www.osha.gov/pls/oshaweb/owadisp.show_document?p_table=STANDARDS&p_id=10051 (accessed Mar. 19, 2005).

2. Joint Commission Resources: *Environment of Care Handbook.* Oakbrook Terrace, IL: Joint Commission on Accreditation of Healthcare Organizations, 2004.

3. Joint Commission Resources: *Infection Control Issues in the Environment of Care.* Oakbrook Terrace, IL: Joint Commission on Accreditation of Healthcare Organizations, 2004.

4. U.S. Department of Labor: Occupational Safety and Health Administration: *Revision to OSHA's Bloodborne Pathogens Standard, Technical Background and Summary.* Washington, DC: OSHA, 2001.

5. American Society of Safety Engineers: *Professional Safety: Needlestick Injuries* 49: Dec. 2004.

6. Joint Commission Resources: Look sharp – Your needlestick prevention program. *Joint Commission Perspectives on Patient Safety* 1: Dec. 2001.

7. U.S. Public Health Service: Centers for Disease Control and Prevention: *Updated U.S. Public Health Service Guidelines for the Management of Occupational Exposures to HBV, HCV, and HIV and Recommendations for Postexposure Prophylaxis.* http://www.cdc.gov/mmwr/preview/mmwrhtml/rr5011a1.htm (accessed Mar. 19, 2005).

8. U.S. Department of Labor: Occupational Safety and Health Administration: *Safety and Health Topics: Tuberculosis.* http://www.osha.gov/SLTC/tuberculosis/index.html (accessed Mar. 19, 2005).

9. U.S. Department of Public Health: Centers for Disease Control and Prevention: *Guidelines for Preventing the Transmission of Mycobacterium tuberculosis in Health Care Settings, 2005 draft.* http://www.cdc.gov/nchstp/tb/Federal_Register/New_Guidelines/TBICGuidelines.pdf (accessed Mar. 19, 2005).

10. U.S. Department of Labor: Occupational Safety and Health Administration: *Occupational Exposure to Tuberculosis; Proposed Rule; Termination of Rulemaking, Respiratory Protection for M. Tuberculosis; Final Rule; Revocation.* http://www.osha.gov/pls/oshaweb/owadisp.show_document?p_table=FEDERAL_REGISTER&p_id=18050 (accessed Mar. 19, 2005).

11. U.S. Department of Public Health: *Centers for Disease Control and Prevention: Guidelines for Preventing the Transmission of Mycobacterium tuberculosis in Health Care Settings, 1994.* http://www.cdc.gov/mmwr/PDF/RR/RR4313.pdf (accessed Mar. 19, 2005).

12. U.S. Department of Public Health: Centers for Disease Control and Prevention: *Legionellosis: Legionnaires' Disease and Pontiac Fever.* http://www.cdc.gov/ncidod/dbmd/diseaseinfo/legionellosis_g.htm (accessed Mar. 19, 2005).

13. U.S. Department of Labor: Occupational Safety and Health Administration: *OSHA Technical Manual, Section III: Chapter 7.* http://www.osha.gov/dts/osta/otm/otm_iii/otm_iii_7.html (accessed Mar. 19, 2005).

14. U.S. Department of Public Health: Centers for Disease Control and Prevention: *Guidelines for Environmental Infection Control in Health Care Facilities.* http://www.cdc.gov/mmwr/PDF/RR/RR5210.pdf (accessed Mar. 19, 2005).

15. Joint Commission Resources: *Infection Control Issues in the Environment of Care.* Oakbrook Terrace, IL: Joint Commission on Accreditation of Healthcare Organizations, 2004.

16. Joint Commission Resources: *Care Delivery and the Environment of Care: A Teamwork Approach.* Oakbrook Terrace, IL: Joint Commission on Accreditation of Healthcare Organizations, 2003.

17. Freije, M. R.: Testing the waters: Facts to consider when deciding whether to sample for *Legionella. Health Facilities Management* 15: May, 2003.

18. American Institute of Architects Academy of Architecture for Health: *Guidelines for Design and Construction of Hospital and Health Care Facilities.* Dallas: Facilities Guidelines Institute, 2001.

19. Kinder, W. E.: *Healthcare Facilities Management Series: Guidelines for Prevention and Control of Legionellae in the Healthcare Environment.* American Society for Healthcare Engineering, Chicago: ASHE, 2001.

20. Freije, M. R.: Pure + Easy: Selecting a Domestic Water Disinfection System. *Health Facilities Management* 16: Sep. 2003.

21. Joint Commission Resources: Legionella contamination curbed at Johns Hopkins Hospital. *Environment of Care News* 7: 4-5, Apr., 2004.

22. U.S. Department of Labor: Occupational Safety and Health Administration: *OSHA's Enforcement Policy to Protect Workers against Glutaraldehyde Exposure.* http://www.osha.gov/pls/oshaweb/owadisp.show_document?p_table=INTERPRETATIONS&p_id=22415 (accessed Mar. 19, 2005).

23. U.S. Department of Labor: Occupational Safety and Health Administration: *Ethylene Oxide.* http://www.osha.gov/pls/oshaweb/owadisp.show_document?p_table=STANDARDS&p_id=10070 (accessed Mar. 19, 2005).

24. U.S. Department of Labor: Occupational Safety and Health Administration: *OSHA Fact Sheet: Ethylene Oxide.* http://www.osha.gov/OshDoc/data_General_Facts/ethylene-oxide-factsheet.pdf (accessed Mar. 19, 2005).

25. U.S. Department of Labor: Occupational Safety and Health Administration: *Medical Surveillance Guidelines for Ethylene Oxide.* http://www.osha.gov/pls/oshaweb/owadisp.show_document?p_table=STANDARDS&p_id=10073 (accessed Mar. 19, 2005).

26. U.S. Department of Labor: Occupational Safety and Health Administration: *Medical Surveillance – Formaldehyde.* http://www.osha.gov/pls/oshaweb/owadisp.show_document?p_table=STANDARDS&p_id=10078 (accessed Mar. 19, 2005).

27. U.S. Department of Labor: Occupational Safety and Health Administration: *OSHA Technical Manual – Section VI: Chapter 1.* http://www.osha.gov/dts/osta/otm/otm_vi/otm_vi_1.html (accessed Mar. 19, 2005).

28. U.S. Department of Labor: Occupational Safety and Health Administration: *Hospital eTool – Healthcare Wide Hazards Module: Glutaraldehyde.* http://www.osha.gov/SLTC/etools/hospital/hazards/glutaraldehyde/glut.html (accessed Mar. 19, 2005).

29. U.S. Department of Labor: Occupational Safety and Health Administration: *Formaldehyde.* http://www.osha.gov/pls/oshaweb/owadisp.show_document?p_table=STANDARDS&p_id=10075 (accessed Mar. 19, 2005).

30. U.S. Department of Labor: Occupational Safety and Health Administration: *Fact Sheet – Formaldehyde*. http://www.osha.gov/OshDoc/data_General_Facts/formaldehyde-factsheet.pdf (accessed Mar. 19, 2005).

31. U.S. Department of Labor: Occupational Safety and Health Administration. *OSHA Technical Manual, Section VI: Chapter 2*. http://www.osha.gov/dts/osta/otm/otm_vi/otm_vi_2.html (accessed Mar. 19, 2005).

32. U.S. Department of Public Health: Center for Disease Control and Prevention: *The Effects of Workplace Hazards on Female Reproductive Health*. http://www.cdc.gov/niosh/99-104.html (accessed Mar. 19, 2005).

33. U.S. Department of Public Health: Center for Disease Control and Prevention: *The Effects of Workplace Hazards on Male Reproductive Health*. http://www.cdc.gov/niosh/malrepro.html (accessed Mar. 19, 2005).

34. U.S. Department of Labor: Occupational Safety and Health Administration: *Anesthetic Gases: Guidelines for Workplace Exposures*. http://www.osha.gov/dts/osta/anestheticgases/index.html (accessed Mar. 19, 2005).

35. U.S. Department of Public Health: Center for Disease Control and Prevention: *NIOSH Warns: Nitrous Oxide Continues to Threaten Health Care Workers*. http://www.cdc.gov/niosh/94-118.html (accessed Mar. 19, 2005).

Chapter 5: Performance Measurement and Worker Safety

THE SAFETY AND QUALITY of care that an organization provides are influenced by worker safety. Workers who enjoy a good work environment, where their safety is of utmost concern to their employers, will make positive contributions to the quality of care provided by the organization. Implementing policies, procedures, and protocols to help preserve the health and safety of workers, such as those discussed in this book, can help organizations improve the health and safety of the workforce and consequently the quality of care provided.

Continuous improvement is critical to the creation of a safe work environment. To continuously improve regarding worker safety an organization must take the following steps (see Figure 5-1):

1. Design a worker safety and health program. This includes the plans, policies, procedures, and controls necessary for a safe work environment. Each of these must be consistent with regulatory requirements and contribute to the provision of quality health care. This serves to set expectations and standardize activities to achieve the desired outcome.
2. Educate employees. The organization's standardized processes should be taught to the organization's staff members so that they become knowledgeable about their role in the environment of care (EC). It is also important in this step to consider contract workers and their knowledge expectations. It is not necessary for everyone to have a complete and thorough understanding of the EC process, but it is important that each person understands his or her individual role as it relates to the EC, both on a routine basis and under emergency circumstances. Education is the critical link between written documentation and proper performance of tasks and activities.
3. Implement Plans. After individuals understand what they have to do to carry out their responsibilities, the plans can be put into action. It is essential that the activities of the staff members in the implementation phase match the written documentation. The organization is expected to fully comply with its own statements of policy and procedure.
4. Measure Success. Putting words into action is only part of the process. It must be followed with an evaluation of how well the plans, policies, and procedures are working; that is, how effective they are at reaching the desired outcome. Each action that the organization

Figure 5-1. The Environment of Care Cycle

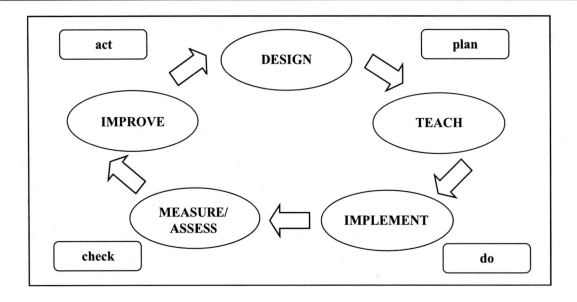

Continuous improvement of the environment of care and worker safety is a continuous cycle.

undertakes should have some means of establishing that it is functioning as planned, some check points to determine if it is on track. Not only is this helpful for new actions but also for existing ones. The policies and procedures that worked last year may not be appropriate now for reasons of new equipment, availability of new information, or identification of a new problem.

5. Continuously Improve. If various measurements indicate that a process is not achieving the desired outcome, or a problem is detected, the organization must improve the process. This could include adjustments, revisions, or complete overhauls. These changes are fed back into the design phase for redevelopment and/or policy and procedure revision, and the cycle begins again.[1]

PERFORMANCE MONITORING IN THE ENVIRONMENT OF CARE

Ongoing monitoring of performance in the environment of care is a necessary function in all care settings. Each of the seven management areas (safety, security, hazardous materials and waste, emergency management, fire safety, medical equipment, and utilities) must be evaluated for actual or potential risk. This means that the organization must look at its processes for managing each area of the environment of care. It must select at least one performance monitor in an area of risk—meaning an area in which it is not doing as well as it should or wants to do. As many monitors as needed may be selected. The organization may not select an issue or process that is the subject of regulatory compliance, as it is already required to monitor that issue. That is, if the organization is not meeting the regulatory standards, it simply must do so. Thus, the organization should instead pick an issue that is problem-prone, or even one that it wants to benchmark to a higher level.

STANDARDS *Joint Commission Standards That Address Performance Measurement in the EC*

➤ EC.9.10, Monitoring Environmental Conditions; EC.9.20, Analyzing Environmental Issues; PI.1.10, Data Collection; PI.2.10, Data Aggregation; PI.2.20, Analyzing Trends
➤ PI.3.10, Data Analysis; PI.3.20, Proactive Program
➤ LD.4.50, Setting Priorities; LD.4.70, Measuring Effectiveness

Chapter 5: Performance Measurement and Worker Safety

At the time of the accreditation survey, it is not necessary to see each management plan with a performance monitor that shows the facility doing perfectly. In fact, if that is what is found, the surveyor will probably ask what else could be measured. Instead, it is more important that the facility is tackling the hard issues. Issues that, when resolved, can have a positive impact on the organization's EC process.

The length of time an organization continues with any given performance monitor varies. Monitoring can continue for a year or more, but if an issue has been corrected, monitoring should be terminated when the organization can reasonably ensure that the correction is being maintained.

The organization should begin the performance monitor selection process by determining what will enable effective management of the EC program. Starting from this perspective will prompt the organization to choose truly meaningful monitors.

Data collection should be considered in the original selection of the monitor. When making the choice, determine how the data are going to be collected from existing sources. If a new system to collect data must be developed and implemented for a given monitor, its chances for success are limited. Some monitors may reflect movement toward an actual target or benchmark, while others follow trends and will never reach a designated end point. An example of this latter type is a monitor that tracks workers' compensation costs. Either type is acceptable.

The concept of performance monitoring carries forward to the management of the EC function in hospital, long term care, ambulatory care, and behavioral health programs. The monitoring data must be reported to and analyzed by the multidisciplinary improvement team (usually called the *safety* or *environment of care committee*). It is suggested that this be done periodically throughout the year. Then, annually, the team must recommend to leadership at least one performance improvement activity in the environment of care. The group makes this recommendation based on the monitoring data and selects a potential performance improvement activity for which administrative and financial support are necessary. Any items that can be easily corrected within the scope and the budget of a department should be corrected by that department over the course of the year.

The organization's leadership will then face the task of prioritizing the EC performance improvement recommendation(s) along with those from the rest of the organization. The decision may or may not be made to implement the EC performance improvement activity. To determine compliance with this requirement, the prioritization process will be reviewed, applying professional judgment. It may be very appropriate that the EC recommendation was not implemented. However, if it is determined that the EC performance improvement recommendation was significant, and a less critical performance improvement project was implemented, an adverse score may be given. For this reason, the individual responsible for managing the EC may want to document the recommendation to leadership and leadership's implementation decision.[1]

Other Performance Measurements

Although performance monitors have specific requirements regarding what can be measured, including actual or potential risk and issues not related to regulatory compliance, that does not imply that measurements related to these topics are not useful and should not be followed.

In fact, an organization will want to know that it is in compliance with all the applicable regulatory issues. For example, it is important to know that the chemical inventory is complete and all the required MSDS have been obtained. These measurements can still lead to improvements.

Ultimately, each health care organization should measure those factors related to worker safety that can give an indication of how the process is working currently and where room for improvement remains.

Performance Measures of Worker Safety

Many of the worker safety issues addressed in this book fall under EC.1.10, Safety Management, or EC.3.10, Hazardous Materials & Waste Management. Some exceptions exist, including references to EC.2.10, Security Management; EC.4.10, Emergency Management; and EC.5.10, Fire Safety.

Remembering the requirements for performance monitoring in general as described previously, the following section will focus on some areas that provide opportunities to monitor or measure performance in worker safety.

Workers' Compensation

Workers' compensation statistics provide data that give an overall picture of worker safety, and tracking them can show improvement or highlight opportunities to improve. For example, workers' compensation costs can reveal trends in worker safety. The dollars spent reflect the number of workplace illnesses and injuries as well as an indication of their severity. This would be a monitor without a defined benchmark or target. No organization will realistically be able to achieve zero cost for workers' compensation. Instead, the organization would follow a trend. Obviously, a downward trend is most desirable, but perhaps holding steady is acceptable under specific circumstances. Certainly no organization wants to see these costs climbing.

Lost work days can be tracked in a similar manner. These directly contribute to the organization's workers' compensation experience rate, hence the insurance premium.

Either of these ways of looking at workers' compensation lends itself nicely to graphical presentation and could be classified as a performance monitor for Joint Commission purposes.

Staff Knowledge

Measurements of staff knowledge regarding worker safety can be measured in a variety of ways. Each staff member is required to attend orientation and education programs to learn how to do his or her job safely. For example, as applicable, employees must be taught what personal protective equipment (PPE) to use, and how and when it must be used. They must learn about the permitting process for confined space entry, and the meaning of locks and tags for electrical safety. They must understand early indications of musculoskeletal injuries, the symptoms of chemical exposure, and the processes to report these. Each chapter of this book contains a host of training requirements.

Monitoring of training could be done by tracking the number of people who attend the designated classes. A more effective assessment would be a measure of staff knowledge. This could be obtained from scores on a test given following a training session. Questions could be asked of staff members during the Joint Commission–required environmental tours, with records of correct and incorrect responses.

Monitoring staff knowledge not only gives the organization a picture of its present performance in worker safety, it clearly identifies where the knowledge gaps are and provides a target for future training. Measures of staff knowledge are applicable as Joint Commission performance monitors.

Other Statistical Measurements

The information provided in this book lends itself to a variety of statistical measurements related to specific topics in worker safety. Included here are some representative areas that can be measured, but there are certainly others. When designing performance monitors for Joint Commission purposes, remember that issues of regulatory compliance should not be used.

Ventilation

Various spaces within organizations have suggested guidelines for air exchanges in those areas. Guidelines found in Table 7.2 of the American Institute of Architects publication, *Guidelines for Design and Construction of Hospital and Health Care Facilities*[2] are commonly used to determine appropriate air exchange rates. It should be noted that these are guidelines for new construction only, and that older facilities may not be able to meet them, nor is that required. Air exchange rates for designated spaces can be measured, tracked, and benchmarked on a regular basis to measure performance.

Noise

Individuals exposed to noise at levels above the action level and other limits described in Chapter Two must have an annual audiogram. An appropriate performance measure would be to record the average hearing loss noted in those audiograms.

Workplace Violence

One of the Joint Commission required functions for security management in health care organizations is to conduct a proactive security risk assessment. One component of that process is an evaluation of the security events that have taken place within the organization. Tracking different types of events, such as thefts, assaults, vandalism, suspicious persons, and so forth provides excellent data to assess the effectiveness of the workplace violence prevention program, and can also be used as performance monitors.

Respiratory Protection

The primary reason for a respiratory protection program in most health care organizations is to reduce exposure to tuberculosis, although there are many other reasons to wear a respirator, as explained in Chapter Three. As fit testing programs are established, an organization could measure the number of individuals who were actually fit tested vs. those who were due for fit testing. Another approach would be those who passed the fit test out of the total number tested. The latter measurement could also be used for performance monitoring, provided that it was an area of risk to the organization.

Chapter 5: Performance Measurement and Worker Safety

Bloodborne Pathogens

As we saw in Chapter Four, all sharps injuries must be recorded in health care organizations. And organizations must work to continually drive down their needlestick injury rates. Monitoring those rates, therefore, is something that must be done. Still, as new engineering controls are available and adopted, it is anticipated that the injury rate will decrease. Measuring the number of needlesticks, therefore, will provide an indication of the effectiveness of worker safety with respect to bloodborne pathogens.

Hazardous Chemicals and Drugs

Many organizations have tried to implement a performance monitor for hazardous materials and waste by counting the number of chemical spills. This is difficult because only the spills that are reported can be counted, and many of them are not reported. Still, this area has ample opportunity for performance measurement by tracking various exposure-monitoring programs.

TIP ▶ A Word of Caution

Some organizations across a variety of industries have embarked on various programs to reduce injury rates by measuring, for example, the number of days without an injury. A variation on that theme would be determining which department has the lowest number of injuries. The department that "wins" this accolade may receive a reward. The danger in this approach is that injuries may go unreported as individuals are discouraged from making reports by co-workers (or themselves) who want to "win." It is suggested that health care organizations look for other ways to reward good performance in worker safety, such as the department where the most people knew the correct answer to the safety quiz.

The Joint Commission and Performance Improvement

The Joint Commission's commitment to performance improvement is not limited to the EC. The issue is pervasive throughout the accreditation standards. While specific applications are listed in many of the more targeted chapters in the accreditation manual, there is the clear expectation that performance improvement must be part of an organization's culture.

A safety culture starts from the top. The organization's leaders provide the framework to plan, direct, coordinate, provide, and improve care, treatment, and services to respond to community, patient, and worker needs, ultimately leading to improved health care outcomes. To reach this goal, effective leadership uses the following processes and tools:

- The governance structure of the organization
- Management responsibility
- Planning, designing, and providing services to support its mission
- Improving safety and quality of care
- Clinical practice guidelines, as applicable
- Teaching and coaching staff

Standards in the Leadership chapter of the accreditation manual support the role of organization leaders in performance improvement.

Putting It All Together

Worker safety is a critical issue to health care organizations. In this era of staffing shortages throughout the industry, health care workers are an extremely valuable resource to be guarded and protected.

Both the Joint Commission and OSHA have pervasive requirements for worker safety in health care organizations. And not only must those requirements be met, but performance records in worker safety must be evaluated and improved where possible.

By continuously improving, organizations have the opportunity to provide an environment that is safe, pleasant and supportive where individuals feel comfortable working and are not worried about their safety. Not only do health care organizations have an ethical obligation to provide such an environment for their employees, but they also can improve the safety and quality of care provided to their patients by improving and enhancing the work environment for their staff.

The picture is clear. The time is now. ■

References

1. Joint Commission Resources: *Environment of Care Handbook.* Oakbrook Terrace, IL: Joint Commission on Accreditation of Healthcare Organizations, 2004.

2. American Institute of Architects Academy of Architecture for Health: *Guidelines for Design and Construction of Hospital and Health Care Facilities.* Dallas: Facilities Guidelines Institute, 2001.

Index

A

Accident investigation, 10
Accreditation surveys
　management plans and, 117
　OSHA compliance issues and, 2, 3
Administrative controls, 11
Airborne contaminants, 19, 31, 36. *See also* Tuberculosis (TB); Ventilation
Airborne infectious isolation (AII) rooms, 31, 96–97
Air exchange rates, 32, 96, 118
Ambulatory care organizations
　EC performance monitoring, 117
　fire safety plan requirement, 27
American Conference of Government Industrial Hygienists (ACGIH), 19, 36, 38, 105
American Hospital Association, 83
American Industrial Hygiene Association (AIHA), 38
American Institute of Architects (AIA)
　air exchange rates, 96
　air handling and ventilation systems guidelines, 31
　dust-control regulations, 38
　Guidelines for Design and Construction of Hospitals and Health Care Facilities, 36, 99, 118
American National Standards Institute (ANSI) standards, 73
American Society of Health-System Pharmacists (ASHP), 111
American Society of Heating, Refrigerating, and Air-Conditioning Engineers (ASHRAE), 31, 36, 96
Anesthetic gas, 107, 109, 111–112
Asbestos, 40–42
　engineering controls for, 42
　materials that may contain, 41
　medical surveillance for exposure to, 41
　OSHA regulations for, 40–42
　personal protective equipment (PPE) for, 42
　staff training and education on, 41–42
　standards (Joint Commission) for, 40
Aspergillus sp., 36
Association for Professionals in Infection Control and Epidemiology (APIC), 38, 83, 95
Audiometric testing, 44

B

Background screenings, 52
Back injuries, 1, 60, 61, 63–64
Behavioral health care organizations
　EC performance monitoring, 117
　fire safety plan requirement, 27
Biological agents, 19, 31
Biological safety cabinets (BSC), 110
Blake Medical Center Voluntary Protection Program, 16–18
Bloodborne pathogens exposure, 87–93
　controls for, 89–92
　exposure control plan, 88–89
　exposure determination, 89
　hepatitis B vaccinations, 92
　infectious agents transmitted through, 88, 89
　opportunities for exposure, 1, 88
　OSHA regulations, 13, 88–89, 92–93
　performance measurements, 119
　personal protective equipment (PPE) for, 74, 89, 91
　recordkeeping of, 22
　response to exposure, 92–93

safer needle devices, 89–90, 91
staff training and education, 93
standards (Joint Commission), 87–88
Bromine for *Legionella pneumophilia* control, 100
Building related illnesses (BRI), 36
Business occupancies, fire safety and, 28

C

Carolinas HealthCare System safety and health program case study, 12–15
Case studies
    Blake Medical Center Voluntary Protection Program, 16–18
    Carolinas HealthCare System safety and health program, 12–15
    Circle Family Care, Inc., mercury cleanup, 20–21
    Duke University Hospital ergonomics, 68
    Florida infectious diseases outbreak, 34
    George Washington University Hospital gas fire emergency, 70–71
    Johns Hopkins Hospital Legionella control and prevention, 102–3
    Kaiser Permanente mold management, 37–40
    Sunnybrook & Women's SARS experience, 32–33
    University of Maryland Medical Center respiratory protection program, 80–82
    Veterans Health Administration ergonomics program, 64–68
    Veterans Health Administration norovirus outbreak, 75–78
    Veterans Health Administration workplace violence, 57–59
Cash-handling areas and violence risk, 51
Centers for Disease Control and Prevention (CDC)
    Guidelines for Environmental Infection Control in Health Care Facilities, 98–99
    mold management program, 38
    risk reduction strategies, 95
    tuberculosis controls, 96, 97
    tuberculosis guidelines, 83, 93, 94
    tuberculosis statistics, 93
Chemicals. *See* Hazardous materials and waste
Chlorine dioxide for *Legionella pneumophilia* control, 101, 102
Chlorine for *Legionella pneumophilia* control, 100, 101, 102
Circle Family Care, Inc., mercury cleanup case study, 20–21
Confined spaces, 25–26
    OSHA regulations, 26
    OSHA training requirements, 13
    staff training and education, 26
    standards (Joint Commission), 25–26
Continuous improvement for worker safety, 115–116
Contractors, hazardous materials requirements for, 21
Contract workers, 10, 11
Control of Hazardous Energy (OSHA), 28
Cooling towers, 100
Copper-silver ionization, 101
Critical incident stress debriefing (CISD), 54
Crosswalk of OSHA topics to Joint Commission standards, 2, 4–5

D

Data collection for performance measurement, 117
Decontamination activities, 78–79
    OSHA regulations, 79
    standards (Joint Commission), 78

De-escalation techniques, 55, 57
Droplet nuclei, 93
Duke University Hospital ergonomics case study, 68
Dust and control measures for, 38, 74

E

EC. *See* environment of care entries; Management of the Environment of Care (EC) standards
Electrical equipment, 28–30
Electrical safety. *See* Hazardous energy and electrical safety
Emergency action planning. *See* Emergency response
Emergency departments, designing for safety, 56
Emergency response
    case study, 70–71
    infectious diseases outbreak case study, 34
    management plan, 2, 68–71, 116
    OSHA regulations, 69
    OSHA training requirements, 13
    respiratory protection program case study, 80–82
    SARS case study, 32–33
    staff training and education, 27, 70
    standards (Joint Commission), 68, 69, 70
Energy control program, 29–30
Engineering controls, 11
Environmental tours requirement, 9, 10
Environment of care committee, 9, 117
Environment of care cycle, 115–116
Environment of Work concerns (OSHA), 2, 3
Equipment maintenance, 11
Ergonomics, 60–68
    case study, 64–68
    controls for, 63–64
    cost of injuries, 60, 61
    ergonomics stressors, 60
    minimal lift environmental program, 63
    musculoskeletal disorders (MSDs), 60
    OSHA regulations, 60, 62, 63
    Patient Assessment Criteria (VA), 66
    patient lifting and, 63–64
    Patient Transfer Algorithm (VA), 67
    program to protect workers, 62–64
    staff training and education, 64
    standards (Joint Commission), 61–62, 63
    statistics on, 60
Escalating behavior signs, training to recognize, 55, 56
Ethylene oxide, 103–107
    characteristics of, 104
    controls for, 105–106
    exposure to, 105
    medical surveillance for exposure, 106
    OSHA regulations, 37, 104
    staff training and education, 106–7
    standards (Joint Commission), 103
Evacuation and exit routes, 69

F

Female reproductive hazards, 108–109
Filtration of air, 31, 32, 33, 96–97
Fire safety, 26–28
    fire extinguisher training, 13
    gas fire emergency case study, 70–71

INDEX

management plan, 2, 116
OSHA regulations, 27
plan requirement, 27
staff training and education, 27
standards (Joint Commission), 26–27
Florida hospitals' infectious diseases outbreak case study, 34
Formaldehyde, 103–107
   as airborne contaminant, 35, 36
   characteristics of, 104
   controls for, 105–106
   exposure to, 105
   medical surveillance for exposure, 106
   OSHA regulations, 104
   staff training and education, 106–107
   standards (Joint Commission), 103
Fungus, 36

G

Gangs, 50–51
Gas fire emergency case study, 70–71
Gastroenteritis outbreak case study, 75–78
General Industry Standards (OSHA), 2, 3
George Washington University Hospital gas fire emergency case study, 70–71
Gloves, 73, 75, 91, 106
Glutaraldehyde, 103–107
   as airborne contaminant, 36
   characteristics of, 104
   controls for, 105–106
   exposure to, 105
   medical surveillance for exposure, 106
   OSHA regulations, 104
   staff training and education, 106–107
   standards (Joint Commission), 103
Guards for machines. *See* Machine guarding
Guidelines for Design and Construction of Hospitals and Health Care Facilities (AIA), 36, 99, 118
Guidelines for Environmental Infection Control in Health Care Facilities (CDC), 98–99
"Guidelines for Nursing Homes—Ergonomics for the Prevention of Muscoskeletal Disorders" (OSHA), 65
"Guidelines for Preventing Workplace Violence for Health Care and Social Service Workers" (OSHA), 52

H

Halogenated agents, 109
Handguns, 50
Handwashing procedures, 90
Hazard communications, 13, 18–21, 107
Hazardous drugs
   controls for, 110–111
   disposal of, 111
   home care settings and, 110
   identification of, 107–108
   medical surveillance for exposure, 112
   OSHA regulations, 107
   performance measurements, 119
   personal protective equipment (PPE) for, 110–111
   spills, 111
   staff training and education, 112
   standards (Joint Commission), 107

Hazardous energy and electrical safety, 28–30
   OSHA regulations, 28–29
   standards (Joint Commission), 28
Hazardous materials and waste, 18–21. *See also* Ethylene oxide; Formaldehyde; Glutaraldehyde
   case study, 20–21
   chemical inventory, 19
   chemical labeling, 19–20
   contractors' requirements for, 21
   decontamination activities, 78–79
   management plan, 2, 116
   "OSHA Best Practices for Hospital-Based First Receivers of Victims of Mass Casualty Incidents Involving the Release of Hazardous Substances", 79
   performance measurements, 119
   Permissible Exposure Limits, 19
   personal protective equipment (PPE) for, 74
   staff training and education, 20
   standards (Joint Commission), 18, 19, 20
   Threshold Limit Values, 19
Hazard reporting system, 9, 10
Hearing conservation, 42–44, 74, 118
HEPA filters, 31, 32, 33, 96–97
Hepatitis B vaccinations, 92
Histoplasma sp, 36
Home care settings
   hazardous drugs and, 110
   violence prevention program, 52
   violence risk factors, 51
Hospitals
   EC performance monitoring, 117
   fire safety plan requirement, 27
   "OSHA Best Practices for Hospital-Based First Receivers of Victims of Mass Casualty Incidents Involving the Release of Hazardous Substances", 79
Hot water recommendations for *Legionella pneumophilia* control, 99, 101, 102
Hot work permits, 27
Housekeeping procedures
   bloodborne pathogens exposure, 91–92
   Sick Building Syndrome (SBS), 35
HVAC systems. *See also* Ventilation
   airborne contaminants, spread through, 36
   Legionella pneumophilia control and, 100–101
   maintenance of, 32, 37
   tuberculosis (TB) contamination, 36
   tuberculosis controls, 96

I

Improvements to environment of care and worker safety, 115–16
Indoor air quality, 31, 37
Indoor air quality program, 37
Injury and illness records, 10–11, 21–22, 55

J

Johns Hopkins Hospital Legionella control and prevention case study, 102–103
Joint Commission. *See also* Standards (Joint Commission)
   partnership with OSHA, 2
   safety, commitment to, 2, 119

K

Kaiser Permanente mold management case study, 37–40

L

Laboratories, fire safety plan requirement, 27
Laundry procedures and bloodborne pathogens exposure, 91–92
Leadership and administration role in safety and health programs, 8–9, 119
Leadership Standards, 4–5, 119
Legionella pneumophilia, 97–103
    case study, 102–3
    characteristics, 98
    controls for, 99–101
    culturing policies, 98–99
    Maryland guidelines, 99
    OSHA regulations, 98
    prevalence of, 97
    risk assessment, 98
    sources of, 98
    staff training and education, 103
    standards (Joint Commission), 98, 99
    surveillance process, 99
    types of, 97
    water treatment options, 100, 101, 102–103
Legionellosis, 97
Legionnaire's Disease, 36, 97
Life Safety Code® (National Fire Protection Association), 27, 28
Lockout/tagout regulations, 28, 29–30
Long term care organizations
    EC performance monitoring, 117
    fire safety plan requirement, 27
    nursing home ergonomics guidelines (OSHA), 62, 63–64, 65
    Veterans Health Administration ergonomics program case study, 64–68
    Veterans Health Administration norovirus outbreak case study, 75–78

M

Machine guarding, 44–47
    guard characteristics, 45–46
    OSHA regulations, 45–46
    OSHA training requirements, 13
    staff training and education, 46–47
    standards (Joint Commission), 45
Management of Human Resources standards, 4–5
Management of Information standards, 4–5
Management of the Environment of Care (EC) standards
    crosswalk of OSHA topics to Joint Commission standards, 4–5
    management plan requirements, 2
    performance measurements, 117
    relationship to General Industry Standards (OSHA), 2, 3
Management of the Environment of Care standards. See also standards (Joint Commission)
Maryland guidelines for Legionella pneumophilia, 99
Material safety data sheets (MSDS), 19
Matrix for safety and health program, 12, 15
Medical equipment management plan, 2, 116
Mentally ill persons, 51
Mercury cleanup case study, 20–21
Minimal lift environmental program, 63
Mold management case study, 37–40
Musculoskeletal disorders (MSDs), 60
Mycobacterium tuberculosis, 36, 93. See also Tuberculosis (TB)

N

N-95 respirator, 81
National Fire Protection Association
    Life Safety Code®, 27, 28
    respiratory protection, 82
Needlestick injuries, 1, 91. See also Bloodborne pathogens exposure
Needlestick Safety and Prevention Act, 88
Negative air pressure, 31, 33
Nitrous oxide, 109, 111
Noise exposure, 42–44, 74, 118
Norovirus outbreak case study, 75–78
Nursing home ergonomics guidelines (OSHA), 62, 63–64, 65
Nursing workforce, aging of, 60

O

Occupational Exposure to Hazardous Chemicals in Laboratories Standards (OSHA), 72–73
Occupational Safety and Health Administration (OSHA)
    crosswalk of OSHA topics to Joint Commission standards, 2, 4–5
    Environment of Work concerns, 2, 3
    General Industry Standards, 2, 3
    "Guidelines for Nursing Homes—Ergonomics for the Prevention of Muscoskeletal Disorders", 65
    "Guidelines for Preventing Workplace Violence for Health Care and Social Service Workers", 52
    Occupational Exposure to Hazardous Chemicals in Laboratories Standards, 72–73
    "OSHA Best Practices for Hospital-Based First Receivers of Victims of Mass Casualty Incidents Involving the Release of Hazardous Substances", 79
    OSHA Technical Manual, 37
    partnership with Joint Commission, 2
    Respirator Medical Evaluation Questionnaire, 81, 83
    Respiratory Protection e-Tool, 23, 82
    safety, commitment to, 2, 119
    Standards for General Industry, 107
    Voluntary Protection Programs, 16–18
    Web site, 42, 81, 107
Occupational Safety and Health Administration (OSHA) regulations
    asbestos, 40–42
    bloodborne pathogens exposure, 13, 88–89, 92–93
    confined spaces, 26
    Control of Hazardous Energy, 28
    cooling towers, 100
    decontamination activities, 79
    electrical equipment, 28–29
    emergency response planning, 69
    energy control program, 29–30
    ergonomics issues, 60, 62, 63
    ethylene oxide, 104
    fire safety plan, 27
    formaldehyde, 104

INDEX

glutaraldehyde, 104
hazard communications, 18–21, 107
hazardous drugs, 107
hazardous energy and electrical safety, 28–29
hearing conservation, 43–44
Legionella pneumophilia, 98
lockout/tagout regulations, 28, 29–30
machine guarding, 45–46
nursing home ergonomics guidelines, 62, 63–64, 65
Permissible Exposure Limits, 19
personal protective equipment (PPE), 72–73, 91
respiratory protection, 79, 80, 81, 82–83
for safety and health programs, 8
security risks, 52, 53
staff training and education, 13
300 Log, 21–22, 55
tuberculosis (TB), 94
ventilation, 30–31
OSHA. *See* Occupational Safety and Health Administration (OSHA)
"OSHA Best Practices for Hospital-Based First Receivers of Victims of Mass Casualty Incidents Involving the Release of Hazardous Substances", 79
OSHA Technical Manual, 37
Ozone for *Legionella pneumophilia* control, 101

P

Patient, definition, 3
Patient Assessment Criteria (VA), 66
Patient lifting and ergonomics, 63–64
Patient Transfer Algorithm (VA), 67
Performance measurement, 115–119
    data collection and analysis, 117
    management plans and, 116–117
    of safety and health programs, 9
    staff knowledge of safety issues, 118
    standards (Joint Commission), 116–117
    statistical measures, 117–119
    workers compensation statistics, 117–118
Permissible Exposure Limits, 19
Permit-required spaces, 25–26
Personal protective equipment (PPE), 71–79
    for asbestos, 42
    bloodborne pathogens exposure, 89, 91
    case study, 75–78
    decontamination activities, 78–79
    formaldehyde, 106
    glutaraldehyde, 106
    for hazard control, 11
    for hazardous drugs, 110–111
    OSHA regulations, 72–73, 91
    OSHA training requirements, 13
    selection of, 73–75
    staff training and education, 75
    standards (Joint Commission), 72, 77
    tuberculosis controls, 97
    use of, 75
Pharmacies and violence risk, 51
Plan for Improvement (PFI), 27
Plumbing system recommendations, 99–100
Pontiac Fever, 97
Positive air pressure, 31

Powered air-purifying respirators (PAPR), 81, 110
Prevention and Management of Disruptive Behavior, 58
Provena Health minimal environmental program, 63

R

Recordkeeping of injuries and illnesses, 10–11, 21–22, 55
Regulated waste disposal, 91–92
Regulatory Assessment Matrix, 12, 15
Reproductive hazards, 108–109
    staff training and education, 112
    standards (Joint Commission), 107
Respiratory protection, 79–84
    case study, 80–82
    ethylene oxide, 106
    fit testing, 83
    formaldehyde, 106
    glutaraldehyde, 106
    hazardous drugs, 110
    maintenance of, 84
    medical evaluation prior to use, 81, 82–83
    OSHA regulations, 79, 80, 81, 82–83
    performance measurements, 118
    seal check, 83
    selection of, 82, 106
    staff training and education, 80–81, 83–84
    standards (Joint Commission), 79, 80
Risk assessment
    Legionella pneumophilia, 98
    requirement for, 10
    security risks, 52–53
    tuberculosis (TB), 95–96

S

Safe Patient Handling and Movement Conference, 65
Safer needle devices, 89–90, 91
Safety
    administration and leadership role in, 1, 119
    Joint Commission commitment to, 2, 119
    OSHA commitment to, 2, 119
    responsibility for, 1–2
    staff role in, 1–2
    standards (Joint Commission), 7–8
Safety and health programs
    accident investigation, 10
    case study, 12–15
    design of, 115, 116
    development of, 7–8
    emergency response management plan, 11
    equipment maintenance, 11
    hazardous materials and waste, 18–21
    hazard prevention and control, 11
    hazard reporting system, 9, 10
    injury and illness records, 10–11, 21–22, 55
    leadership support for, 8–9
    OSHA regulations, 8
    OSHA training requirements, 13
    participation in, 8, 9
    performance monitoring of, 9
    risk assessment requirements, 10
    staff training and education, 11–12, 116
    standards (Joint Commission), 15, 17

workplace analysis, 10
Safety committee, 9, 117
Safety hot line, 9
Safety liaison, 9
Safety management plan, 2, 116
Safety officers, 1, 7, 8–9
Safety policies and procedures, 1, 9
Safety report form process, 9
SARS case study, 32–33
Screening for TB, 96
Security management plan, 2, 52, 53, 116
Security risk assessment, 52–53
Self-contained breathing apparatus (SCBA), 82, 84
Severe Acute Respiratory Syndrome (SARS) case study, 32–33
Sharps handling and disposal, 90, 91
Shift changes and violence risk, 51
Sick Building Syndrome (SBS), 34–36
Society for Healthcare Epidemiologists of America (SHEA), 95
Staff TB screening, 96
Staff training and education
    anesthetic gas, 112
    asbestos, 41–42
    bloodborne pathogens exposure, 93
    de-escalation techniques, 55, 57
    emergency response, 27
    emergency response management plan, 70
    ergonomics program, 64
    escalating behavior signs, training to recognize, 55, 56
    ethylene oxide, 106–107
    fire safety, 27
    formaldehyde, 106–107
    glutaraldehyde, 106–107
    guarded machinery use, 46–47
    hazardous drugs, 112
    hazardous materials and waste, 20
    indoor air quality, 37
    Legionella pneumophilia, 103
    lockout/tagout procedures, 30
    measurement of, 118
    OSHA requirements, 13
    performance measurements, 118
    permit-required spaces, 26
    personal protective equipment (PPE), 75
    reproductive hazards, 112
    respiratory protection, 80–81, 83–84
    safety and health programs, 11–12, 116
    tuberculosis risks, 97
    violence in the workplace, 54–56
Standard Precautions (Universal Precautions), 89
Standards (Joint Commission)
    anesthetic gas, 107
    asbestos, 40
    bloodborne pathogens exposure, 87–88
    confined spaces, 25–26
    crosswalk of OSHA topics to Joint Commission standards, 2, 4–5
    decontamination activities, 78
    emergency response planning, 68, 69, 70
    ergonomics issues, 61–62, 63
    ethylene oxide, 103
    fire safety, 26–27
    formaldehyde, 103
    glutaraldehyde, 103
    hazardous drugs, 107
    hazardous energy and electrical safety, 28
    hazardous materials and waste, 18, 19, 20
    hearing conservation, 42
    Legionella pneumophilia, 98, 99
    machine guarding, 45
    performance measurement, 116–17
    personal protective equipment (PPE), 72, 77
    recordkeeping, 21
    reproductive hazards, 107
    respiratory protection, 79, 80
    safety, 7–8
    safety and health programs, 15, 17
    tuberculosis (TB), 94, 95
    ventilation, 30, 31, 39
    violence in the workplace, 51, 52, 59
    worker safety, 2
Standard threshold shift (STS), 44
Star status, 17
Statement of Conditions™ (SOC), 27
Strength/Witness/Opportunity/Threat Analysis (SWOT), 13
Sunnybrook & Women's SARS experience case study, 32–33

T

Tampa General Hospital infectious diseases outbreak case study, 34
300 Log, 21–22, 55
Threshold Limit Values, 19
Tuberculosis (TB), 93–97
    contamination through HVAC system, 36
    controls for, 96–97
    OSHA regulations, 94
    prevalence of, 93, 95
    prevention and control programs, 95–96
    recordkeeping of tests, 22
    respiratory protection for, 83
    staff training and education, 97
    standards (Joint Commission), 94, 95
    transmission of, 95

U

Ultraviolet germicidal irradiation (UVGI), 97
Ultraviolet light for *Legionella pneumophilia* control, 101
United States Environmental Protection Agency (US EPA), 38
Universal Precautions (Standard Precautions), 89
Universal Precautions for Violence, 54
University of Maryland Medical Center respiratory protection program case study, 80–82
Utilities management plan, 2, 116

V

Ventilation, 30–40
    airborne contaminants, 19, 31, 36
    air exchange rates, 32, 96, 118
    building related illnesses (BRI), 36
    case studies, 32–34
    case study, 37–40
    engineering controls for, 36–37
    filtration of air, 31, 32, 33, 96–97

formaldehyde, 105–106
general dilution ventilation, 111
glutaraldehyde, 106
indoor air quality, 31
indoor air quality program, 37
OSHA regulations, 30–31
performance measurements, 118
pressure relationships, 31–32, 97
Sick Building Syndrome (SBS), 34–36
standards (Joint Commission), 30, 31, 39
waste anesthetic gas (WAG), 111
Veterans Health Administration ergonomics program case study, 64–68
Veterans Health Administration norovirus outbreak case study, 75–78
Veterans Health Administration workplace violence case study, 57–59
Violence in the workplace
    case study, 57–59
    categories of, 49
    characteristics, 49–50
    controls for, 53–54
    critical incident stress debriefing (CISD), 54
    definition, 49
    examples of, 50
    OSHA training requirements, 13
    performance measurements, 118
    prevention program development, 51–57
    risk factors, 50–51
    staff training and education, 54–56
    standards (Joint Commission), 51, 52, 59
    statistics on, 50
Volatile organic compounds (VOCs), 35, 36
Voluntary Protection Programs (OSHA), 16–18
    case study, 16–18
    star status, 17

W

Waste anesthetic gas (WAG), 109, 111–112
Waterborne bacteria. *See Legionella pneumophilia*
Water intrusion and mold management (WIMM) program, 38–40
Water treatment for Legionella pneumophilia control, 100, 101, 102–103
Web sites
    Occupational Safety and Health Administration (OSHA), 42
    OSHA safety and health topics, 107
    respiratory protection program, 81
    Safe Patient Handling and Movement Conference, 65
Worker safety
    improvements to environment of care and, 115–116
    prevalance of injuries, 1
    standards that address, 2
    workers compensation statistics, 117–118
Workers compensation statistics, 117–118
Work practice controls, 11